MY QUEST

MY QUEST

THE
Chronicle-Record
OF MY QUEST FOR A LIFE, DELIVERANCE, AND REDEMPTION

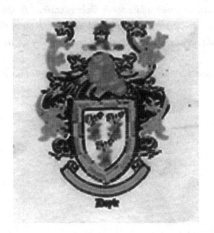

AN AUTOBIOGRAPHICAL SKETCH OF A COMMON MAN WHO, PLAGUED BY SCHIZOPHRENIA AND OTHER PROBLEMS, BATTLES TO GAIN (AND SOMETIMES REGAIN) A LIFE WORTH LIVING—AND TO FIND DELIVERANCE FROM DEMONS AND ENJOY ULTIMATE REDEMPTION; A TRUE ACCOUNT, AN EVOLVING PERSONAL PROFILE, AND A SAGA SPANNING SIXTY-FIVE YEARS PLUS.

RONALD F. DOYLE

iUniverse, Inc.
Bloomington

MY QUEST
The Chronicle-Record of My Quest for a Life, Deliverance, and Redemption

iUniverse books may be ordered through booksellers or by contacting:

iUniverse
1663 Liberty Drive
Bloomington, IN 47403
www.iuniverse.com
1-800-Authors (1-800-288-4677)

ISBN: 978-1-4620-4275-3 (sc)
ISBN: 978-1-4620-4276-0 (ebk)

Printed in the United States of America

iUniverse rev. date: 10/07/2011

EDITOR'S NOTE:

In order to assure privacy, the names of many living individuals mentioned in this book have been omitted, shortened, or changed. Also, the names of client companies are protected except where public announcements have been made after the completion of a project.

ACKNOWLEDGEMENTS

I, the author, wish to acknowledge the many people who have helped me write this book, have encouraged me along the way, or have aided me in my life's struggle. Especially, I acknowledge the ever-present assistance of my mother, the late Irma M. Doyle, who was a true source of unconditional love to the very end of her life. She also took the time and made the effort to proofread and criticize line-by-line the entire book that had been written before her death. Her contribution to this story and story-telling was monumental. This book is dedicated to her memory lovingly.

Also, I want to thank from the bottom of my heart the many people who have reviewed all or parts of the book, rendered their advice and impressions, and encouraged me to continue. Especially I want to thank my cousin, Tom Doyle, and my aunt, the late Elsie Brumbaugh, for their careful reading and input.

THANK YOU ONE AND ALL.

PREFACE

This book is the end product of forty years of scrapbooking, photo album creation, journaling and other writing. Especially in the last twenty years I have developed this book by writing several editions, each one updating, expanding on, or contracting an earlier version.

My first scrapbooks date from when I was still in high school. At that time I was convinced I was beginning to write the story of a "great man to be." Of course, my plan didn't work out. God had other plans. What ultimately emerged is the autobiography of an uncommonly common man who, plagued by schizophrenia and other problems, battled to live a life worth living, to be delivered from enemies, and to ultimately experience redemption. It traces my life from conception to my sixty-fifth birthday—a saga of sixty-five years plus. This book is my principal written legacy to my family and relatives present and future.

MY CROSS: SCHIZOPHRENIA

Schizophrenia is defined by Webster's Dictionary as "a mental disorder characterized by indifference, withdrawal, hallucinations, and delusions of persecution and omnipotence, often with unimpaired intelligence: a more inclusive term than *dementia praecox* avoiding the implications of age and deterioration." Schizophrenia, that mysterious brain disorder, has been the main limiter of my life's activities—afterward ranked everything else. Schizophrenia often robs its victims of part of their intellectual capabilities and sometimes even blocks out reality for days or weeks at a time. The 'voices' one hears scare other people who hear about them. But, how much more they scare the patient, the one hearing the voices!

Schizophrenia is a major impediment to employment across the boards (from the boardrooms to the trenches) as *stress*—often just job stress after a month or two—activates the chemical imbalance in the brain which causes schizophrenic symptoms making work activity impossible or of poor quality. Employers, familiar with the illness' effects, disdain to hire schizophrenics for any job with responsibilities that could pay a living wage. As a result, the unemployment rate for people with schizophrenia seeking employment approaches one hundred percent typically everywhere in the U.S. For those who can get jobs job security is non-existent, promotions are unusual. And 'poor judgment' on-the-job stemming from schizophrenic lapses often causes friction with other employees as well.

Lack of good job prospects coupled with poor judgment periods (including errant behavior) make schizophrenics disadvantaged as a choice for most meaningful relationships including but not limited to marriage and parenthood. Few eligible partners want a close relationship with a schizophrenic—and in some states having such a relationship is a crime! Additionally, since the root cause of the illness is genetic and passed on through the genes, children of a schizophrenic are more likely to be schizophrenic themselves once they reach fifteen to twenty-five years of age, the age at which schizophrenia is usually first diagnosed.

To add insult to injury, the disease carries a stigma: that the individual himself or herself is responsible for having the condition. Some suggest that the condition is 'chosen'. Clearly no one would choose to have this illness. Others suggest that it results from "sin". While all schizophrenics have committed sins, so has everyone else. And, whereas one percent of the general adult population is schizophrenic, seven percent of the general adult population are convicted criminals. Most schizophrenics—despite experiencing periods of dimmed intellect and bad judgment—have had no trouble with the law.

Then again, bad parenting, particularly by the mother, is often blamed as the culprit. But, in my family both my brothers have led exemplary lives as overachievers. We all three had the same mother. And my mother was a living saint who loved me very much.

As a result of all the before mentioned, most schizophrenics I know of tend to live single lives, have few friends, and usually practically no money. And because of the stigma as well as variability of mental acuity, find themselves marginalized by society year after year. Most of our lives are both depressing and dull.

On the positive side, schizophrenia is not fatal . . . Or, is it? About 15% of people who get the illness succeed in committing suicide. The principal reason seems to be to 'escape from the madness'. On a more hopeful note, 1 in 5 schizophrenics eventually cease to evidence any symptoms and are able to return to a normal life. When this occurs it is usually about 10 years after the last psychotic break experienced. And for the 80% who remain ill, requiring heavy doses of expensive medication to function, the medications are much improved with fewer side effects than 40 years ago. The atypical anti-psychotic drugs such as *risperdal* (and others) have made life easier for most still effected by the illness. Public educational campaigns have increased awareness of the real causes of schizophrenia and reduced stigma while increasing understanding.

Yet even here there is a problem: as an ill person becomes higher functioning to the point where he or she appears to be "well" even to the schizophrenic, when he or she is not, it is difficult to get continued funding. My own feeling is that only a trained psychiatrist can tell if a person has passed through the crises and is fit to work again or not. It's been my experience that some psychiatrists are more aware of the problems faced by schizophrenics than others and more willing to speak up for their patients. To the best of my abilities I have not depended on the disability insurance system. Instead, because I was higher functioning and prodded by my father I tried and continue to try harder to work and support myself. But commercially acceptable work eventually became impossible for me as it does in most cases of this illness barring remission.

MY MISSION: POSITIVE REALISM

As my life has been largely a struggle against schizophrenia and its consequences, my mission in this book is to "take a bite out of the dog which bit me" by busting negative stereotypes and reducing stigma by detailing the positive accomplishments of my life, the life of a man who has battled schizophrenia for forty plus years. While some critics may argue that glossing over the negativity leads to an untrue picture, I say that I only wish to emphasize the positive. Yes, negatives were there but I view my life as more than half filled with positivity, not nearly half empty of accomplishment—a contrast in perspectives. I celebrate many partial victories ignoring shortfalls (which were largely due to the illness in one way or another).

A secondary intent of this approach is to encourage schizophrenics (and other mentally ill people) as well as families of these people that there is no need to give up on life simply because of an adverse diagnosis and condition. While not to trivialize the severe disadvantages of schizophrenia, life still beckons all to embrace it. It is just that to do so is now tougher. But, with faith in God, the help of understanding family and friends, and struggle, the battle can be won to an extent needed to have many happy periods. People are just tougher than they at first think they are.

MY LIFE

The book reviews my life as I lived it chronologically. Chapters one and two visit the first 36% of my life, a time before the onset of schizophrenia, and the events of those years of my youth. Chapters three and four review my working career troubled but not yet disabled from schizophrenia. It covers the second third of my life before age 62. Chapters five and six give a detailed look at my life after the government found me to be 'totally disabled'. This last third of my life before age 62 I struggled unsuccessfully to regain a financially productive life. Schizophrenia was the principal culprit. But I did manage to be of use to my family—principally my mother in her final years on Earth.

I realize that I am incompetent to render a judgment on myself in this book. That Judgment will come from Christ as I pass on into Eternity. At that time my "handicap" will be properly considered and my hopes and prayers noted. At the time of Judgment we are assured we'll each get "what we deserve" and "many who were first will be last, and many who were last first".

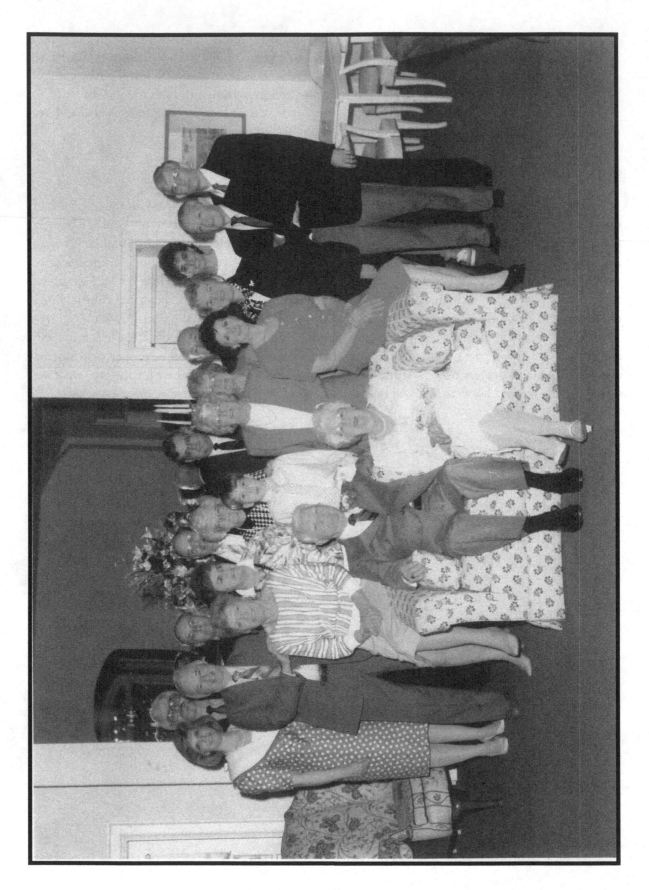

CHAPTER ONE

THE FAMILY

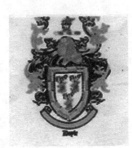

I came from a good family. My father's side was Irish-American from way back. It was a large family, almost a "clan." My mother's side were Austro-Hungarians of (back then) relatively recent immigration. I had two brothers, one older and one younger.

PROLOGUE

These are the generations who preceded me:

The marriage of Vincent Leo Doyle and Irma Ann Milisits took place on April 29, 1939 at Blessed Sacrament Roman Catholic Church in Newark, NJ. It united the Doyle clan with the Milisits family.

THE DOYLES

On my father's side, the Irish . . . From way back our "ancestral homeland" had been New Jersey. My ancestors had a large dairy and produce farm in what is now the City of Kearny, Hudson County, New Jersey. Family legend says it was a plum from the then new U.S. Government to illustrious forbearers, taken from Tories departing for elsewhere after the American Revolution.

MY PATERNAL GRANDPARENTS

My grandfather was Thomas Doyle, who had a dairy farm in Kearny. A Democrat who refused to join a Republican sponsored union (of milk producers) he found his barn torched by persons unknown in the highly Republican town. He quickly resorted to running a vegetable wagon and had a second job later as a park policeman. "PRODUCE" was the product and motto of his small company.

He was a man of few words but much action.

My grandmother was Mary Donnelly, also of Kearny. This Doyle-Donnelly union produced 13 pregnancies, 10 children 9 of whom lived to adulthood. She spent her time taking care of the kids and died young of cancer at 47. My grandmother died in 1933 and my grandfather in 1947 of diabetes.

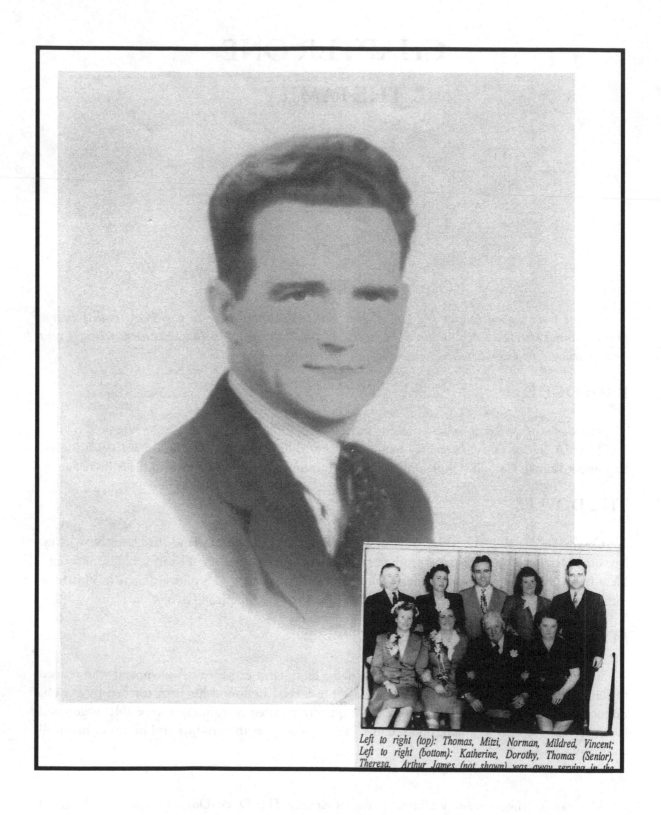

Left to right (top): Thomas, Mitzi, Norman, Mildred, Vincent;
Left to right (bottom): Katherine, Dorothy, Thomas (Senior),
Theresa. Arthur James (not shown) was away serving in the

DAD: VINCENT LEO DOYLE

Dad was born in 1909 in Kearny. He started a career with E. I. DuPont in 1925 at the age of 16. Beginning at the Arlington (NJ) Works as a tradesman and later general foreman, he accepted a transfer to Washington (WV) Works just outside of Parkersburg, WV, in 1956, where he was central shops foreman (over the trades) and later overseer of outside contractors brought on the plant site to do multiple internal contract jobs.

Dad retired in 1974 after 47 years of service. Until he died (December 1993), he still lived in West Virginia and was an elderly booster of the State. Although registered Republican, he had an independent outlook, often favoring certain Democratic politicians.

MY UNCLES

Uncle Tom: He was born in 1905. He was a band leader, later a policeman in the park force, and even later ran his own gardening business. Married twice, he had two children. He lived all of his life in New Jersey (Kearny and later the Jersey Shore). He died in 1988.

Uncle Norman: He was born in 1913. A U.S. Army captain during the 30's, he later became a prominent union leader and Democratic politician in Kearny and Hudson County, New Jersey. He gained the greatest visibility of any of the surviving DOYLE-DONELLEY offspring. He had two children by his first wife. Widowed young, he married again. He died in 1973?

Uncle Jim: My godfather was born in 1924. A World War II Marine Corps combat veteran (Pacific Theatre), he was a tradesman and later a construction superintendent. On the road often, he maintained a home in New Jersey and was active in local politics. He had one child by his first wife, Mary. Also widowed young, he remarried. He lived with his second wife until his 2005 death.

MY AUNTS

Aunt Theresa: "Aunt Tessy" was born in 1903. She married Arty Grimes, a nightclub entrepreneur. Together they lived in Kearny, NJ and had 3 children. She died in 1964.

Aunt Mitzi: Born in 1907, she married Norman Riley, also a nightclub entrepreneur and small businessman. They lived in Nutley, NJ and had one child. She died in 1965?

Aunt Katherine: She was born in 1911. She married Gerald Carney, a school teacher. They lived in Harrison, NJ and had one child. She died in 1980.

Aunt Dot: She was born in 1918. She married Charlie Carr. Both worked decades for RCA and lived in Lyndhurst, too. They had no children, but Charlie had one son from a previous marriage. She died in 1980.

Aunt Mildred: "Aunt Milly" was born in 1921. A grand old lady . . . never married. She worked decades for Western Electric while living in Kearny and retired to the Jersey Shore area where she lived until she died in 1999.

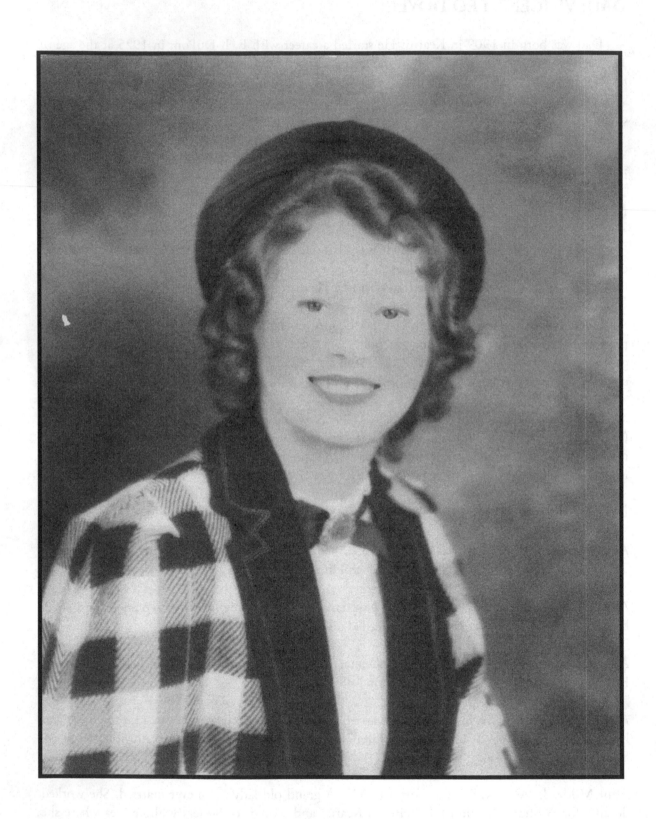

THE MILISITSES

On my mother's side, the Austro-Hungarians . . .

MY MATERNAL GRANDPARENTS

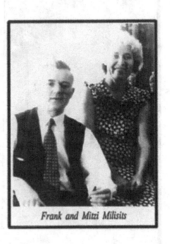

Frank and Mitzi Milisits

My maternal grandparents were both immigrants to America in the decade or so before World War I broke out in Europe. My grandfather, Frank Milisits, was a Croatian living in Hungary (from Santpeterfa, Hungary) during the time of the old Austro-Hungarian Empire. My grandmother, Mitzi Tansits, was an Austrian who emigrated from Güssing near the current border with Hungary.

My maternal grandfather and grandmother met over here, having both immigrated through Ellis Island. My grandfather was a tailor. My grandmother took care of their two children.

MOM: IRMA M. DOYLE

Mom was born in 1910 in New York City, but was reared in Scranton and Northampton, PA and Newark, NJ. Before marriage, she worked 13 years in the audit section of The Prudential Life Insurance Co. in Newark, NJ. Afterward, she was a housewife and mother to us three boys. She lived in West Virginia until going to the nursing home just before her 2007 death.

UNCLE ED: Born in 1917, he was during World War II a U.S. Army paratrooper (European Theatre). He worked later two careers: as a Bell Labs efficiency technician (New Jersey), and as a hotel-motel owner and operator (Florida). Married with no children he retired young, and lived in Florida with his wife, Elsie, until his death (1995).

THREE SONS

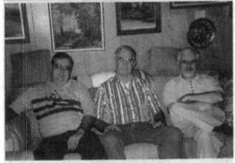

Ron, Vince, and Tim

VINCENT
Vince was born in 1941. A graduate of the University of Dayton (B.S./M.S.-Engineering), he was a captain in the U.S. Army during the Vietnam era (stationed on the Korean DMZ). He returned to become an engineer at General Electric. Married to Margie Smith, they had three children and live in the suburban Ohio.

TIMOTHY
Born in 1950, Tim is a graduate of the University of Dayton (B.S./M.S.-Engineering) and holds a law degree from Wayne State University. He began as an engineer at Ford Motor Co. in Detroit in 1973 and soon progressed into management positions. Married to Kathy Cole, they had one adopted child. They now are retired and live in Michigan.

RONALD
Please read on . . . .

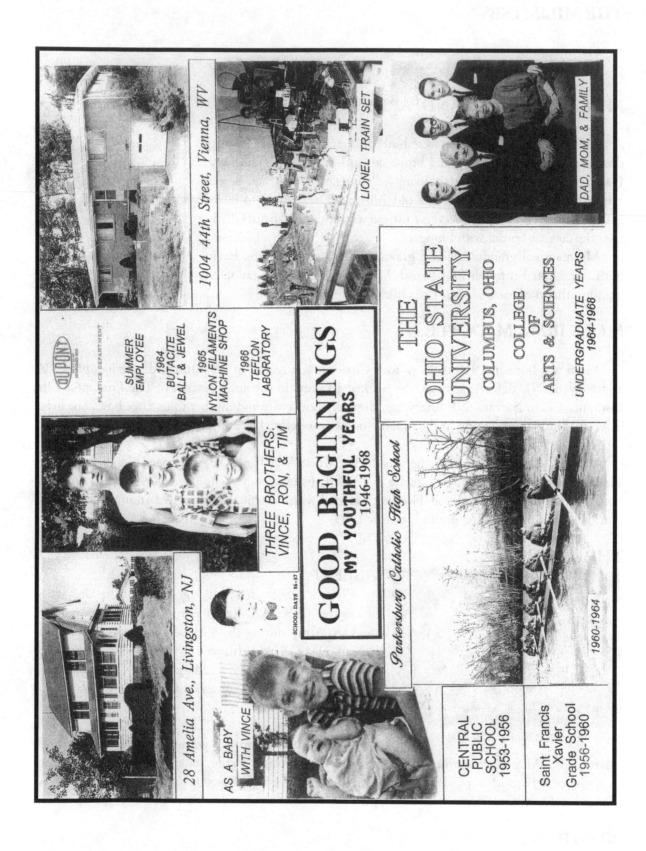

1004 44th Street, Vienna, WV

LIONEL TRAIN SET

DAD, MOM, & FAMILY

DUPONT

PLASTICS DEPARTMENT

SUMMER EMPLOYEE

1964 BUTACITE BALL & JEWEL

1965 NYLON FILAMENTS MACHINE SHOP

1966 TEFLON LABORATORY

THE OHIO STATE UNIVERSITY
COLUMBUS, OHIO

COLLEGE OF ARTS & SCIENCES

UNDERGRADUATE YEARS 1964-1968

THREE BROTHERS: VINCE, RON, & TIM

GOOD BEGINNINGS
MY YOUTHFUL YEARS
1946-1968

SCHOOL DAYS 56-57

28 Amelia Ave., Livingston, NJ

AS A BABY

WITH VINCE

Parkersburg Catholic High School

1960-1964

CENTRAL PUBLIC SCHOOL 1953-1956

Saint Francis Xavier Grade School 1956-1960

CHAPTER TWO
GOOD BEGINNINGS

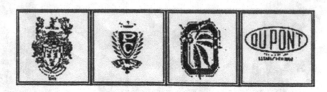

I grew up in Livingston, NJ in a lower middle class Catholic home and had a relatively normal childhood generally. At nine, my father being transferred, I relocated with my family to West Virginia. There I later completed grade school, graduated from high school, and went off to college (OSU).

My first years at OSU were generally uneventful and normal. Toward 1968, among other things, the military draft for the Vietnam conflict began to close in on me . . .

MY CHILDHOOD

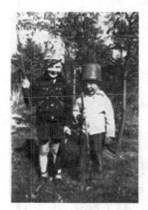

THE FORMATIVE YEARS IN THE SUBURBAN NYC AREA

I was born May 2, 1946 at 2 PM EDT in a hospital in East Orange, NJ. My mother was 36, my father was 37. My older brother's name was Lynn (a name he later renounced in favor of "Vince"). My childhood friends were Jimmy Casius, and Susan and Kathy Denton. All were neighborhood children. Brother Tim joined the family in 1950, completing the trio of the Doyle boys from Livingston. My childhood was extremely happy, very active, very normal, and relatively favorably remembered by myself and others. When I began school (public school) I began to grow socially.

Home, 28 Amelia Avenue, was my first school. I learned to eat, use the toilet, walk, talk, and generally grow "in wisdom and strength". I was baptized in the Roman Catholic Church, and was a member of St. Philomena's parish in Livingston. I attended public kindergarten. The following year I was enrolled in Central Public School in Livingston, which was located just at the foot of Amelia Ave. where we lived. It was a short walk to school and I came home many times for lunch on school days. I remember playing soccer frequently at recess time. I was a good student.

My parents' house where I lived was a two-story house with a full basement and attic. There were two large garages in the back of the property. The yard was large consisting of two 150'x 168' lots side by side. I was neither spoiled nor deprived of toys and other possessions, and I had my very own bedroom in which to store most of them. I played "cowboys and Indians," "cops and robbers," and "soldier" very much with the other kids in the neighborhood dressed in costume.

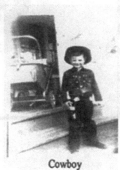

Cowboy

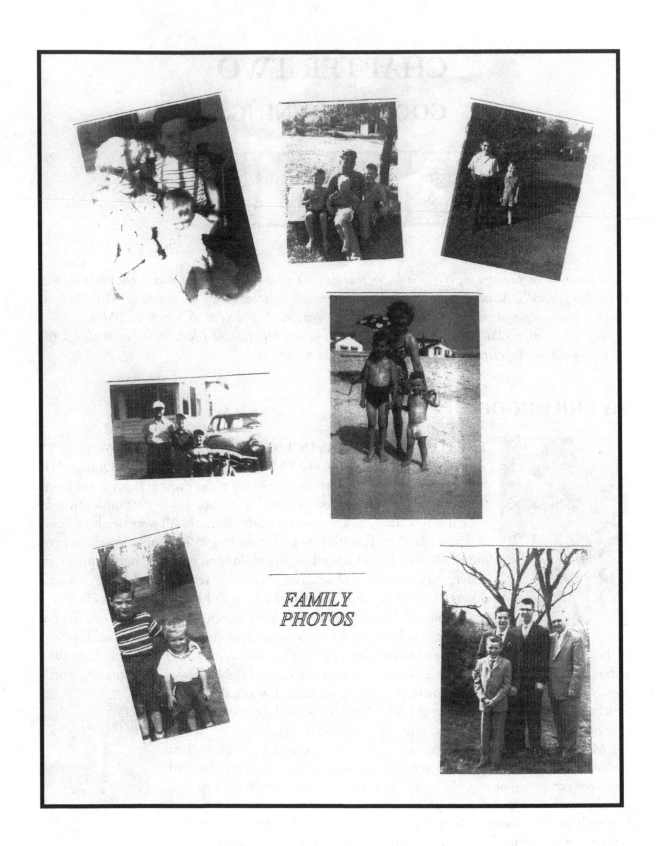

FAMILY
PHOTOS

I had few medical problems as a child, aside from the usual childhood diseases: mumps, scarlet fever, and measles. I did, however, have a hernia from an early age. It limited my physical activities somewhat and I had to wear a truss. It resulted in my parents being somewhat excessively protective of me in my early years because of the handicap. While we lived in New Jersey, my father was a general foreman at E. 1. DuPont in Arlington. He had started as a laborer in 1926 and rose through the ranks. He made a modest but steady income. Mom, who from 1926 to 1939 had worked in the audit section at The Prudential in Newark, stayed at home to raise the children. The family's financial circumstances were such that we could not often afford the luxuries of life, but never wanted for the necessities.

THE TRANSFER

In 1956, the family moved to West Virginia because my father accepted a transfer to Washington Works there, the Arlington plant being closed down. When I left New Jersey, I sadly left friends behind. I also left behind frequent visits from my extended family members. I was then nine years old.

MY EARLY ADOLESCENCE IN VIENNA, WEST VIRGINIA

At DuPont in the Parkersburg area Dad was the foreman in charge of Central Shops (all the trades) for a number of years. Our standard of living improved somewhat during these years as the cost-of-living was lower in West Virginia than it had been in New Jersey and Dad's salary grew also. Difficulties on the job, reportedly with "the bastards" (With job experience, I now know what he was talking about back then). It kept Dad preoccupied with his job and keeping an income coming in. Eventually, however, things worked out and Dad returned to a more sublime mood.

Once we had moved to West Virginia, I was enrolled in St. Francis Xavier Grade School in Parkersburg, and was taught mostly by nuns. I took the city bus to and from school and made the one-half mile walk to and from the bus stop every school day. Often, (literally) running late, Mrs. Packard, a kind soul, would come by in her car and pick up stragglers like me (who missed the bus) and take us to school.

In grade school, I quickly excelled in studies (like most of the children from New Jersey, we were ahead of the locals educationally). In junior high, I played basketball and was considered good at that sport at that time: I grew tall earlier than the others. One buddy of the era was Steve Pulaski, with whom I competed academically in junior high and whose parents had similarly transferred in from New Jersey. After the eighth grade, he went away to the seminary to study for the priesthood, but later chose not to become a priest.

In West Virginia, we lived at a rented house at 802 33rd Street in Vienna until the "new house" that my parents designed and had built was completed. That "new house" is located at 1004 44th Street in Vienna. It is at the end of a short dead-end street, and overlooks a creek valley (Pond Run) 60 feet below. Excavation dirt from the foundations was pushed into an adjoining side yard (which is part of the property) and leveled making a significant open space before the drop-off into the creek valley.

In West Virginia, I owned not only my own bike, which I valued for the mobility it gave me, but also a Lionel train set which preoccupied me many a day after school—designing layouts, and whole villages to go with the layouts. I occupied the greater part of the back basement with my train board and equipment.

Emotionally, however, especially after the move to West Virginia, I became more withdrawn (although denying it). I most often did not seek involvement with others my age, but accepted it as the price of developing my skills, talents, and mind. I was not part of the in-crowd often. Rather, I was a loner more than not. However, I had friends and was largely accepted and/or tolerated by my peers at that time.

HIGH SCHOOL
HAPPY DAYS: AN ERA OF RED, WHITE, AND BLUE

In high school, my friendships developed from and centered about my school, I was narrowly anchored, having only Catholic friends, and dating only Catholic girls.

I remember that I got along fairly well with the boys. I dated one of the girls from freshman year through much of junior year. I "played the field" afterwards, taking a beautiful young lady to the prom senior year.

I had no close friends, however. My own family was closest to me.

Freshman year at the then new high school (Parkersburg Catholic), I found myself mixed in and competing with new young people who recently graduated from St. Margaret Mary Grade School. New friendships and new adversaries were made. At first, I was popular, was elected class treasurer, and I quickly gained the lead academically. Soon, however, my abilities at basketball waned, (strategies proved mentally difficult for me as my body was not coordinating with my mind), and my popularity declined as some made fun of me, becoming nicknamed as "the idiot".

Sophomore year was difficult. But in junior year I got involved in the crew (rowing) team, made varsity crew and regained an acceptable social status, all the while continuing to do well in studies. During the following summer, I represented the school at a Week In Washington with our area U. S. Congressman, then Ken Hechler (D-WV), and at the Rotarians' World Affairs Institute in Morgantown. Particularly the Week in Washington was a positive experience.

During both junior and senior year I went on road trips with our crew coach, and the rest of the

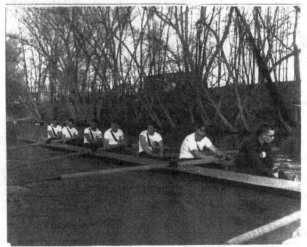

crew team. Among the places we rowed were: Culver Military Academy on Lake Maxinkuckee, Chicago on the Lincoln Canal, Washington DC on the Potomac, and Philadelphia on the Schuykill. We also rowed locally on the Ohio and Muskingum Rivers. We were West Virginia state champions in 1964 (we beat PHS, the only other in the state then). The crew racing experience was another of the more positive experiences of my early years.

I was elected class president senior year, replacing another, who had gotten himself in temporary disfavor with the school officials. I was a benign and uninspiring leader, however. My sergeant-at-arms ran most of the meetings from the back of the classroom clueing me what to say at the front. I was also in the cast of "The Mouse That Roared," a play presented at PCHS and also at Morgantown. Moreover, I was also a member of the German language group. Senior year, I was ultimately named class valedictorian and got to give a speech at graduation.

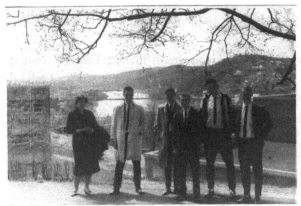

Frau Grev and German language students (including me) at Morgantown

Otherwise, in high school, I was mostly into having a nice wardrobe and a selectivity of clothes for all occasions. I also learned to drive my dad's car, which I borrowed frequently for dates, social occasions, and sports events.

Dad continued to work at DuPont. My first job was as a caddy at the Parkersburg Country Club during the summers. I also had a paper route (a gift from a departing friend) for about a year delivering in the mornings *The Parkersburg News* sometime during my junior and senior years in high school.

EARLY COLLEGE
SUMMERS AT DUPONT AND SCHOOL YEARS AT OSU

Before departing for college, my Dad took me on a short vacation up to New Jersey to visit with my Uncle Norman. He took us all out to a New York nightclub where I watched a show starring Barbara Streisand.

Upon return, I worked full-time one summer at DuPont (as part of their summer employment program for sons and daughters of employees) on the Ball & Jewel (material reprocessing) cutter in Butacite Works.

Off to Ohio State after my first summer at DuPont, I lived on campus in Stadley Hall, a student dorm, sharing a small room with two other guys.

I quickly made friends at OSU, in the dorm and on campus. But, these friends did not last . . . except for Bill Flanigan, who tried steadfastly through my undergraduate years to keep a responsible and respectable Irish Catholic relationship going with me.

Interested in the military programs on campus and initially believing I was or soon would be fit and sold on the notion that the Vietnam intervention was necessary (the Gulf of Tonkin Resolution had been passed by Congress in August), I volunteered for the Naval Reserve Officers Training Corps at

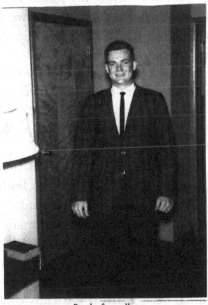

Ready for college...

OSU—and "signed on the dotted line". But my parents whose consent I sought refused to permit it. They just did not want two sons in the military at the same time during a time of conflict until more other families sent their sons or additional sons. My brother, Vince, was an officer in the U. S. Army stationed in Korea at the time.

I worked the following summer at DuPont in the Nylon Filaments shop as a painter.

I "improved" my housing status sophomore year by living off campus at a student rooming house, there finding temporary friendship with a small group of people who were my roommates. My first roommate, however, left school and I went with my second roommate into a cozy little apartment on an alleyway a block or two away. My second roommate, Don had a pet Kingfisher snake that he let roam free around the apartment. Don also left school at the end of the quarter. They never kept in touch with me afterwards though.

I did also spend quite a bit of time sophomore year at OSU Newman Hall (where I attended Mass, often listening to the priests there talk about the events of the times. (Those to whom I talked to tended to be liberal, even radical, and dissuaded me from joining or organizing support for the Vietnam War policy.) Dissuaded from supporting the policy, I was persuaded into being against it. I almost joined SNICC (Student Non-violent Coordinating Committee, an anti-Vietnam War (radical) organization) through a priest, but a brief telephone conversation with one (anonymous) female member/recruiter turned me off on them, and them on me. I wasn't buying what they were selling.

I attended lectures at the Newman Center. the contents of one "history of the Vietnam War" (given by an OSU history professor), I parroted into an easily written English composition (2-page essay credit in English class. I got an "A" on the paper and a mildly sarcastic note from my female teacher (who I listened to because I discerned beforehand that she seemed to be a 'good Democrat') "Have you ever heard of treason?" she wrote. (This really was not what I was about!)

Pretty quickly afterwards, because of their undermining support for my generation grappling with the question of serving in this war, I drifted away from the OSU Newman Club, the Catholic Church, and many other people . . . I'd try to figure things out for myself . . . and talk with others.

Summer before my junior year, I worked at DuPont's Teflon labs. It was the best job I had at DuPont. (A few years later, however, much of that building was blown away in a Teflon explosion that broke windows in Parkersburg, several miles away. Six people, some I knew, were killed or injured.)

Junior year, I lived first at a private dorm off campus. Uncharacteristically, I *almost* punched out one of my randomly-chosen roommates there—he had been meanly tirading for a long period of time against me and I just got tired of being picked on. But, he talked me out of it, agreeing to try to get along better in the future. We did get along OK afterwards for the duration of our common lodgings.

Between junior and senior school years, during the summer, I worked on campus in the work-study program. It was the last fairly clearheaded pleasant times I would have for quite awhile.

Senior year, I lived with some prelaw students on South Campus. However, there I was quickly cast aside somehow as emotionally needy and "strange". I *was*. For, by now the footings under me an all of my collegiate cohorts was starting to get shakier: LBJ had abolished student deferments and America's involvement in Vietnam's civil war was unexpectedly heating up . . .

It seems, also because of the times in America as well as my personal situation, that while during junior year, I had few friends except superficial ones, senior year I was developing more friction with people than friendships. Social relationships were starting to deteriorate some. On the negative side, dates were few and inconclusive . . . my principal lady friend being from "down-home" and a "buddy." I had joined no student or civic organizations of any kind in Columbus or OSU, nor was I motivated or invited to join any during my college years.

On the positive side, I had joined no radical organizations. And, by March was accepted in the graduate school geography program. Academically, I had ground through course after course with A's and B's, and a C here and there until Spring 1968.

During this period, two addresses were my principal possessions: my parents' home address where I stayed registered for voting, the draft, and summer living; and my school address which changed often; along with a few clothes from home.

My status, in retrospect, if I had one, was that I was a normal all-too-honest, detail-oriented, fair, clearheaded, older boy not yet become a young man—just slightly romantic, slightly intellectual . . .

I tried to quietly by myself devise alternative sets of plans depending upon the contingencies presented to me by the future. I began to investigate details. But, I was soon to learn the hard way that some things totally unexpected can happen, and, simply stated, *cannot be planned for* . . .

APPENDIX

APPENDIX

HEALTH DEPARTMENT, ORANGE, N. J.

CERTIFICATE OF BIRTH

I, as Registrar of Vital Statistics, of the City of Orange, in the County of Essex, and State of New Jersey, do hereby certify that the following is a true copy from the Birth Records in my office:

PLACE OF BIRTH

County of Essex, State of New Jersey

City of Orange

No. St. Mary's Hospital

ADDRESS OF MOTHER
Street Address
or R.F.D. Number   28 Amelia Avenue,

City or Borough   Livingston, N.J.
If outside City or
Borough limits, name
Township of Residence

FULL NAME OF CHILD   RONALD   FRANK   DOYLE

SEX	Twin or Triplet	If so, born 1st, 2nd, or 3rd	Months of Pregnancy	Is mother married to father of child?	Date of birth
Male			9	Yes	May 2 19 46

FATHER
FULL NAME   Vincent Leo Doyle

COLOR OR RACE   White   AGE AT TIME OF THIS BIRTH   37

BIRTHPLACE   New Jersey

Usual occupation ...Sheet Metal Smith.................

Industry or Business ....

Children born to this mother:
How many other children of this mother are now living?............1
How many other children were born alive, but are now dead?.............

How many children were born dead?.............

MOTHER
FULL MAIDEN NAME   Irma Ann Milisits

COLOR OR RACE   White   AGE AT TIME OF THIS BIRTH   36

BIRTHPLACE   New York

Usual occupation ...Housewife..................

Industry or business ....

Was a Blood Test for Syphilis made during pregnancy?   Yes | Date Specimen Taken 11/46

What Preventive for Ophthalmia Neonatorum was used?   Agno$_3$ 1%

I hereby certify that I attended the birth of this child who was born alive at.................... 2:44 P. .....m., on the date above stated.

Filed .... May 9 46   Attendant   Dr. Chas. R. Walsh

Registrar .... W. M. Brien, M.D.   Address ....Livingston, N.J.

Corrections and Additions

IN TESTIMONY WHEREOF, I have hereunto set my hand and seal of the Health Department of the City of Orange

on this 9th day of May A. D., 1946

This record is not authentic unless it contains the imprint of the Official seal of the office of the Registrar and unless it is free from alteration of any kind.

Registrar of Vital Statistics

Form 1—3-45-5M

GRADE SCHOOL

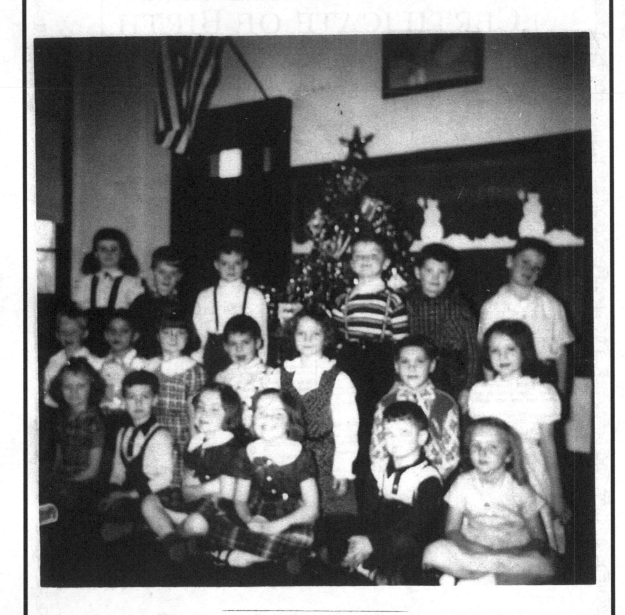

CENTRAL PUBLIC SCHOOL
LIVINGSTON, NJ
1955?

Diocese of Wheeling
Office of Schools

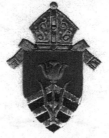

This is to Certify that

Ronald Doyle

Being of Good Christian Character
and having satisfactorily completed in

Saint Francis Xavier School

the Course of Study prescribed for
the Elementary Schools by the Diocese
is awarded this

DIPLOMA

Rev. Daniel M. Kirwin
SUPERINTENDENT OF SCHOOLS

Sr. M. Alfreda, P.C.J.
PRINCIPAL

Parkersburg, W. Va.
May, 1960

John B. O'Reilly
PASTOR

HENRY GRATTAN STUDIOS
EAST ORANGE, N.J.

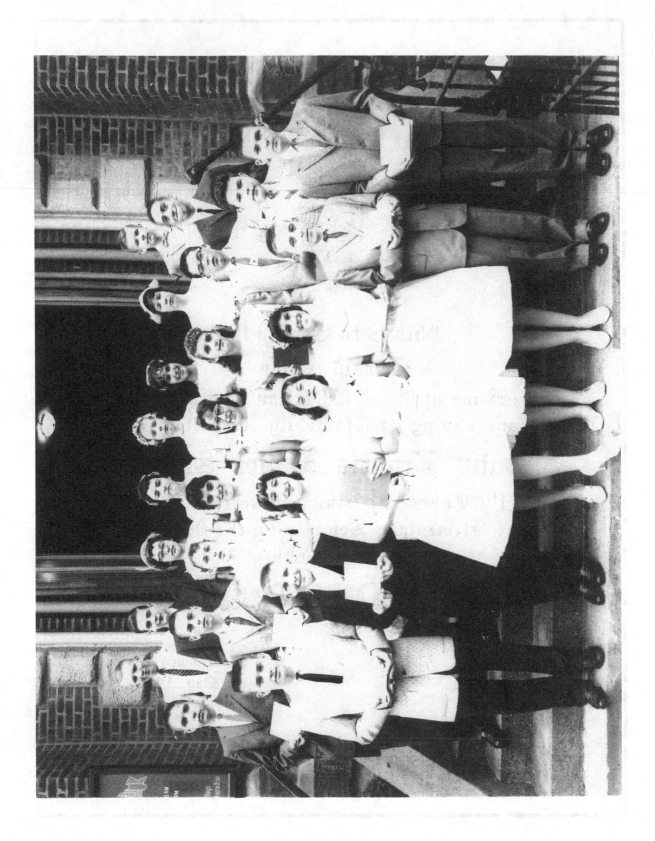

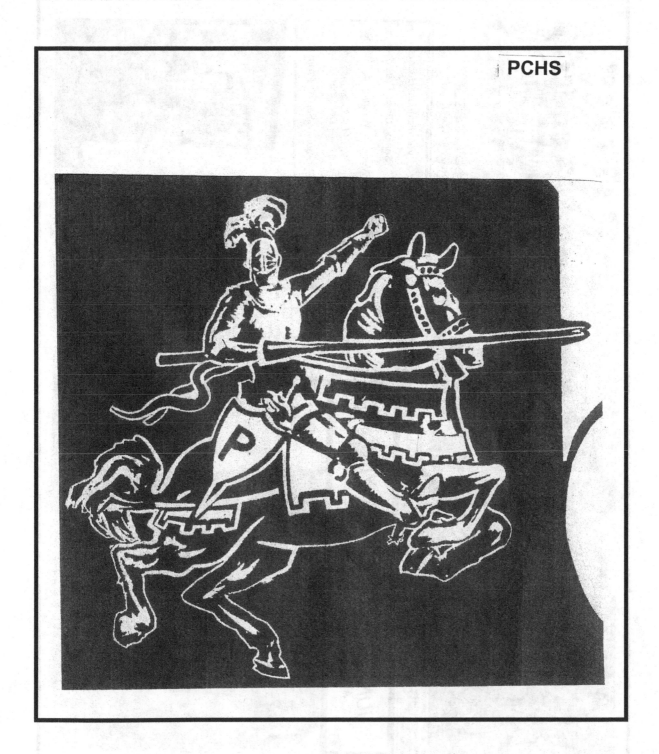

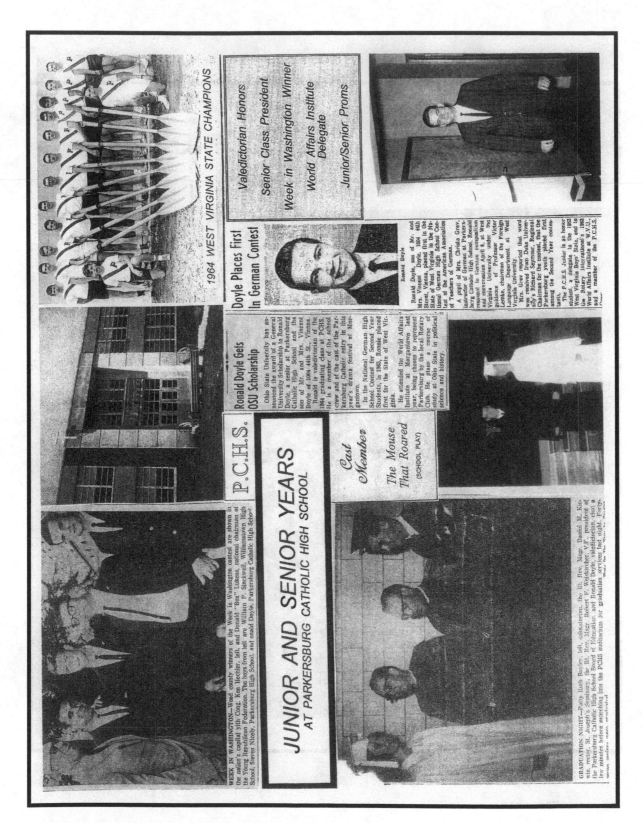

1964 WEST VIRGINIA STATE CHAMPIONS

Valedictorian Honors

Senior Class President

Week in Washington Winner

World Affairs Institute Delegate

Junior/Senior Proms

Doyle Places First In German Contest

Ronald Doyle

Ronald Doyle, son of Mr. and Mrs. Vincent Doyle, 1004 44th Street, Vienna, placed first in the State of West Virginia in the National German High School Contest of Teachers of German.

A pupil of Mrs. Christa Grey, instructor of German at Parkersburg Catholic High School, Ronald engaged in German composition and conversation April 6, at West Virginia University under the guidance of Professor Victor Lemke, chairman of the Foreign Language Department at West Virginia University.

Mrs. Grey reported that word was received from Duke University's Richard Seymour, Regional Chairman for the contest, that the Parkersburg youth placed first among the Second Year contestants.

The P.C.H.S. Junior is an honor student, a delegate to the 1963 West Virginia Boys' State, and to the Rotary International's 1963 World Affairs Institute at W.V.U. and a member of the P.C.H.S. Crew.

Ronald Doyle Gets OSU Scholarship

Ohio State University has announced the award of a General University Scholarship to Ronald Doyle, a senior at Parkersburg Catholic High School and the son of Mr. and Mrs. Vincent Doyle of 1004 44th St., Vienna.

Ronald is valedictorian of the 1964 graduating class at PCHS. He is a member of the school crew and of the cast of the Parkersburg Catholic entry in this year's drama festival at Morgantown.

In the National German High School Contest for Second Year Students, in 1963, Ronnie placed first for the State of West Virginia.

He attended the World Affairs Institute at Morgantown last year, being chosen to represent Parkersburg by the local Rotary Club. He plans a course of study at Ohio State in political science and history.

P.C.H.S.

JUNIOR AND SENIOR YEARS
AT PARKERSBURG CATHOLIC HIGH SCHOOL

Cast Member

The Mouse That Roared
(SCHOOL PLAY)

WEEK IN WASHINGTON—Wood county winners of the Week in Washington contest are shown in the nation's capital with Cong. Ken Hechler, left, and Donald "Buz" Lukens, national chairman of the Young Republican Federation. The boys from left are William P. Stockwell, Williamstown High School, Steven Nicely, Parkersburg High School, and onald Doyle, Parkersburg Catholic High School.

GRADUATION NIGHT—Patty Ruth Bayley, left, salutatorian; the Rt. Rev. Msgr. Daniel M. Kinwin, rector, St. Joseph's Seminary; the Rt. Rev. Msgr. Robert F. Weisheicher, V.F., president of the Parkersburg Catholic High School Board of Education and Ronald Doyle, valedictorian, chat a few minutes before marching into the PCHS auditorium for graduation services last night. Forty-...

KEN HECHLER
4TH DISTRICT, WEST VIRGINIA

STAFF ASSISTANTS:
CARLA HINKLE
NANCY J. LEVERICH
ROBERT R. NELSON
VIRGINIA SKEEN

—PLUS ANY VOLUNTEER
HELP WE CAN GET!

COMMITTEE:
SCIENCE AND ASTRONAUTICS

ROOM 1507, NEW HOUSE OFFICE BLDG.
TEL.: CAPITOL 4-3121, EXT. 3452

HUNTINGTON, W. VA., OFFICE:
ROOM 219, POST OFFICE BLDG.
TEL.: 523-6000

PARKERSBURG, W. VA., OFFICE:
239 COURT SQUARE
TEL.: 428-6789
MRS. ROBERT SIMMONS
IN CHARGE

Congress of the United States
House of Representatives
Washington, D. C.
May 21, 1963

Ronald Frank Doyle
1004 - 44th Street
Vienna, West Virginia

Dear Ron:

It is an honor to inform you that the independent board of judges has selected you as a winner of the 1963 Week in Washington contest.

In order to select the week you are to spend in Washington, please let me know by return mail the dates between June 1-September 1 when you cannot come to Washington. We will then inform you definitely of the week you are scheduled to be here. We are arranging to have the winners leave by train on Saturday evening, arriving in Washington on Sunday morning, after which you will have an opportunity to attend church services in Washington. At the end of the week, you will be leaving Washington by train on Saturday morning, arriving home on Saturday evening.

As soon as we work out your schedule of the week you are to come to Washington, we shall send you full details of the trip and what to plan for and expect. We will send you a round-trip rail coach ticket just before you come to Washington. You will be staying, rent-free, in a comfortable home at 631 G St., S. E., where the telephone number is LIncoln 4-2126. Rev. and Mrs. David Kirk will be living in the house for the summer and will chaperone the group.

At the beginning of the week, you will be given $20.00 in cash to defray food expenses. You might bring a little extra money to cover any entertainment or souvenirs, as this will not be provided for, although this is not necessary. Towels and linens will be provided.

During one week, four or five girls will be here at the same time, and the following week four or five boys will be spending the week here. We are certain you will have a wonderful week here in Washington. We look forward to hearing from you just as soon as possible, and then we will mail additional details.

Your servant in Congress,

Ken Hechler

PARKERSBURG **ROTARY CLUB**

CHARTERED 1919   PARKERSBURG, WEST VIRGINIA

March 27, 1963

Mr. Ronald Doyle
1004 - 44th Street
Vienna, W. Va.

Dear Ronald:

We are most happy to invite you as a representative of your fine Parkersburg Catholic High, at the World Affairs Institute at Morgantown, April 19 and 20.

Unfortunately, our Rotary Club was not permitted to take as many of our students this year as we would like, and hence, we are limited on our participation to five students. For your information, the four from Parkersburg Senior High are David Couch, Michael Matheny, Sherry Corbitt, and Chris Mentzer. You five will be leaving Parkersburg on early Friday morning, the 19th, and having a most wonderful time the rest of that day, and up to and including Saturday afternoon. My good wife has agreed to be chaperon and chauffeur.

We feel that the World Affair Institute is going to have an exceptionally fine curriculum of study this year. Included is the Common Market, United Nations in Africa, Conflict between Russia and Red China, Unrest in South America and other International Problems. Our club will be your host and will take care of all expenses as far as transportation, registration and meals commencing Friday evening and Saturday breakfast, also your lodging which will be at the Hotel Morgan.

We will be in touch with you early in that week to ascertain the best departure time and port of embarkation. We do hope you can join us and we would like to have your answer at your earliest convenience on your acceptance.

Sincerely,

R. E. Mentzer

President
Parkersburg Rotary Club

REM/ls

CRUSADER

Vol. IX No. 2   Parkersburg Catholic   Nov. 1963

IN MEMORIUM

The students of P.C.H.S. mourn with the rest of the nation and the world the passing of the late President of the United States, John Fitzgerald Kennedy.

The late President was a vigorous, dynamic leader, a devoted servant to all the people, and an exemplary Catholic man. He was particularly close to us because of his many efforts to help youth and to revitalize and rededicate the American people to the fulfillment in fact of the ideal of freedom.

Although the man is dead, his principles live on and I hope that the spirit of liberty reawakened in the people shall never again be tempted to sleep.

The President said, "Ask not what your country can do for you, but what you can do for your country." It seems that this was a call to all people, but particularly youth, to be good citizens, spirited with self-sacrifice for the general good. Let us not fail to answer this call to which our beloved John Kennedy gave the last full measure of his life. Let us continue with "renewed vigor" to prepare ourselves to be able as he was able to meet new challenges to our national welfare, for soon the responsibility for meeting these challenges will be our own.

Ronald Doyle--Senior Class President

The Road Not Taken
by Robert Frost

Two roads diverged in a yellow wood,
And sorry I could not travel both
And be one traveler, long I stood
And looked down one as far as I could
To where it bent in the undergrowth;

Then took the other, as just as fair,
And having perhaps the better claim,
Because it was grassy and wanted wear;
Though as for that the passing there
Had worn them really about the same,

And both that morning equally lay
In leaves no step had trodden black.
Oh, I kept the first for another day!
Yet knowing how way leads on to way,
I doubted if I should ever come back.

I shall be telling this with a sigh
Somewhere ages and ages hence:
Two roads diverged in a wood, and I--
I took the one less traveled by,
And that has made all the difference.

IN TRIBUTE

John Fitzgerald Kennedy was a martyr. He didn't die on a fiery cross or in a lion's den, but he was a martyr for the cause of peace and love among men.

Our President has been killed by a hate so strong that the bullet could not have been stopped by all the Secret Service and policemen in the world. The men could not be expected to keep Mr. Kennedy safe from all angles. Their theory has always been that the main protective force was the decency of the American people. Friday, November 22, 1963 proved that something had happened to that decency.

Let us hope and pray that John F. Kennedy's martyrdom will help us out of the pit of anger and hate into which we have fallen.

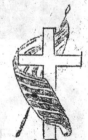

"Ask not what your country can do for you, but what you can do for your country." These were the words spoken by our late President, John F. Kennedy, at his inauguration on that cold day in January, 1961. Let these words inspire each of us to the highest loyalty to God and our country.

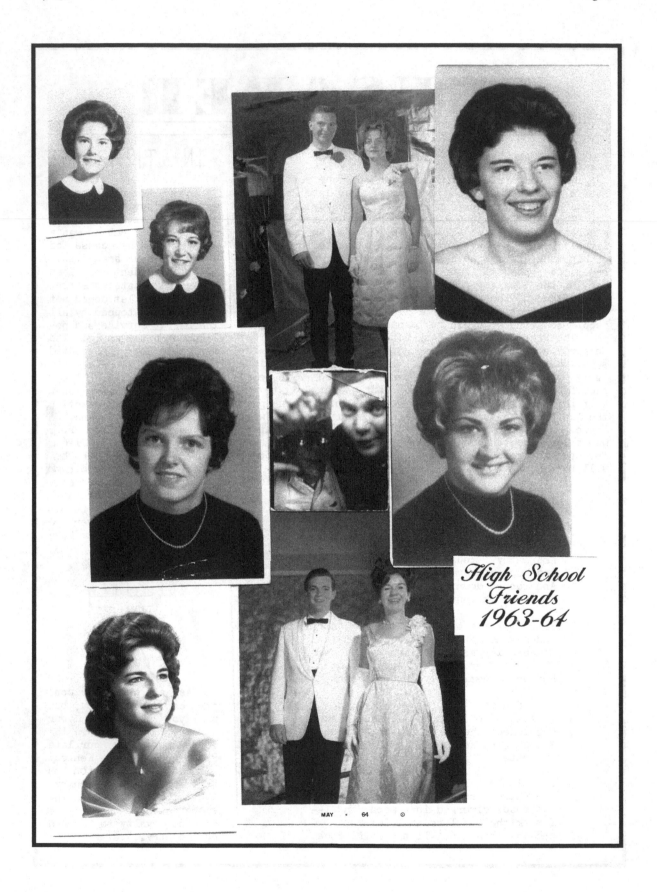

High School
Friends
1963-64

MAY · 64 ⊙

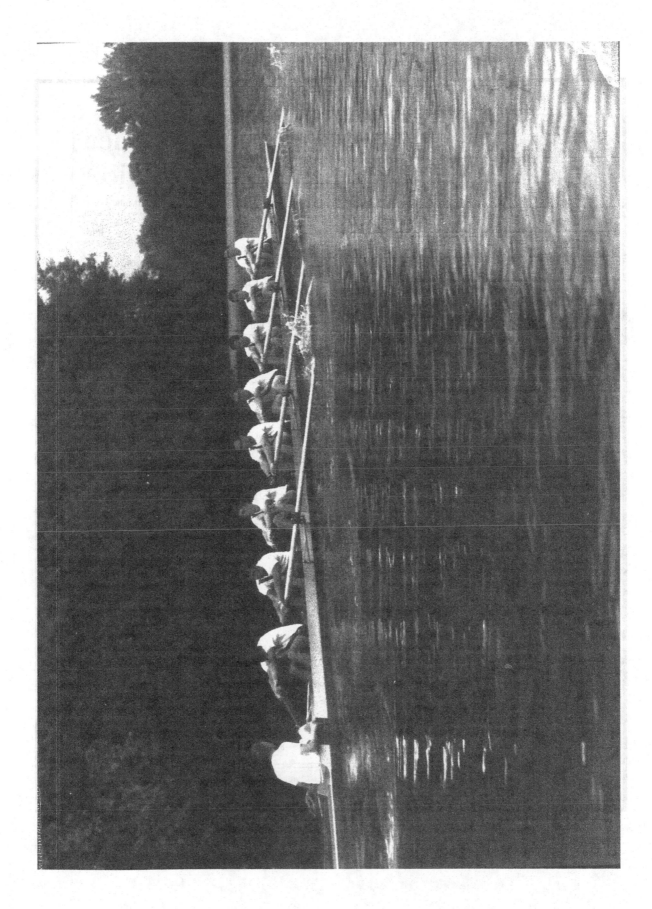

Crusader Crew To Row in Washington

Parkersburg Catholic's varsity crew will leave this morning for the nation's capital where the Crusaders will compete in the Northern Virginia High School championships on the Potomac River Saturday afternoon.

Coach Bruce Allen Herbert said Thursday the Crusaders will compete in the jayvee division against such powers as Washington & Lee High, George Washington, Hammon and St. Andrews. Washington & Lee has been the national scholastic crew champion for the last five years.

Slated to make the trip are oarsmen Don Brown, Matt Santer, Rich Litwinko, Carl Swartzmiller, Bob Albright, Dave Pierson, Dick Schaffer, Ron Doyle, Mike Flanagan, Dan Murphy and Coxswain Joe Tucker.

Accompanying the crew will be Coach Herbert, Dr. Oliver Brundage, Ralph Flanagan and the Rev. Robert Park.

Crusader Oarsmen Beat Culver Twice

CULVER, Ind.—Parkersburg Catholic's varsity crew powered to a one-half length victory over Weber High School of Chicago and to a three-length decision over the Culver Military Lightweight crew in a race held on Lake Maxinkuckee here Saturday.

Conditions were far from ideal on the big lake. The water was rough and the crews rowed into a headwind over the one-mile course.

Coach Bruce Allen Herbert said the Crusaders started at 40 strokes an dsprinted ito a half-length lead. The Blues settled at 34 in the body of the race and finished with a strong 39.

"I was very pleased with the boys," Herbert said. "They did just exactly what we had planned and won easily. I was particularly proud of our new coxswain, Jim Sheridan."

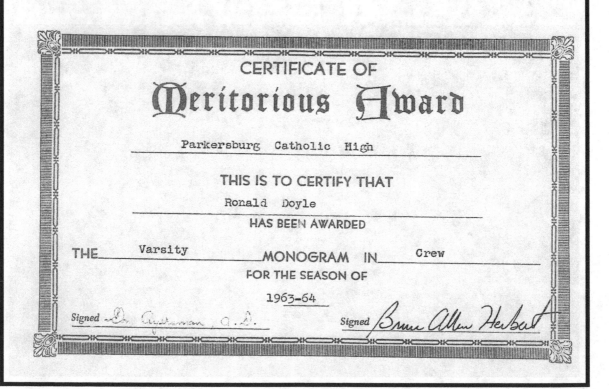

CERTIFICATE OF

Meritorious Award

Parkersburg Catholic High

THIS IS TO CERTIFY THAT

Ronald Doyle

HAS BEEN AWARDED

THE ___Varsity___ MONOGRAM IN ___Crew___

FOR THE SEASON OF

1963-64

Signed _D. Cushman, A.D._   Signed _Bruce Allen Herbert_

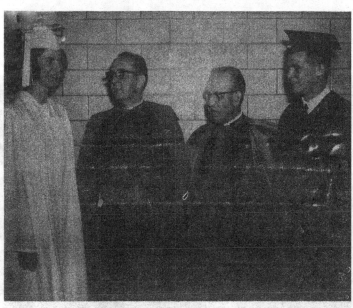

GRADUATION NIGHT—Patty Ruth Bayley, left, salutatorian, the Rt. Rev. Msgr. Daniel M. Kirwin, rector, St. Joseph's Seminary, the Rt. Rev. Msgr. Robert F. Weiskircher, V.F., president of the Parkersburg Catholic High School Board of Education, and Ronald Doyle, valedictorian, chat a few minutes before marching into the PCHS auditorium for graduation services last night. Forty-seven seniors were graduated.
Photo for The News by Headley

PROGRAM

Processional — POMP AND CIRCUMSTANCE .... Elgar
Orchestra

Fourth Degree Knights of Columbus
Graduates of 1964
Faculty

OUR NATIONAL ANTHEM

Invocation .... Rt. Rev. Msgr. Daniel M. Kirwin
Rector, St. Joseph's Seminary

Salutatory .... Miss Patty Ruth Bayley

YOU'LL NEVER WALK ALONE .... Rodger, Hammerstein
Class of '64

PRAISE TO THE LORD .... Gesangbuch
Glee Club

Valedictory .... Mr. Ronald Doyle

CLIMB EV'RY MOUNTAIN .... Rodgers, Hammerstein
Class of '64

Address .... Rt. Rev. Msgr. Robert Weiskircher
President PCHS Board of Education

PRESENTATION OF DIPLOMAS .... Rt. Rev. Msgr. Robert Weiskircher

PSALM 150 .... Louis Lewandowski
Glee Club

PRESENTATION OF AWARDS .... Rev. Francis Scheuerman

Benediction .... Rev. Thomas Fitzgerald

ALMA MATER .... P.C.H.S. Students

Recessional .... Orchestra
American Federation of Musicians, Local 259

Miss Kathryn Sell, Miss Pamela Hall

GRADUATES

Patty Ruth Bayley
Barbara Ann Brundage
Sherry Michele Brock
Shelia Yvonne Coury
Leslie Ruth Cummins
Linda Kay Dye
Barbara Lynn Engle
Martha Louise Eyermann
Margaret Ann Foreman
Marian Jean Franz

Marjorie Ann Glaser
Kathleen O'Donnell Heyel
Genie Marita Higginbotham
Cora Mary Higgins
Martha Susan Kroger
Sharon Louann Lanum
Linda Suzanne Lamb
Lucy Anne Liotti
Helen Anne McDonough
Patricia Ann Sheets

Thomasina Kathryn Shipman
Mary Martha Strain
Janet Kay Tresino
Linda Kay Weser
Sandra Ann Weser
Terry Anne Williams
Martha Elaine Workman

Robert Reinhard Albright
Donald Arthur Brown
Ronald Frank Doyle
Michael David Flanagan
Michael Robert Hattman
James Bernard Hayhurst
Warren Thomas Huxley
Zachary Taylor Jones
David Sassin Joseph
James William Lauer

Richard Allen Litwinko
John Samuel Lutz
William Robert Meintel
Kevin Henry Oliphant
Ralph Wendel Sadie
Mathew Paul Santer
Joseph Michael Schaffer
Richard Paul Schaffer
Joseph Carroll Tucker
John Robert Whitlatch

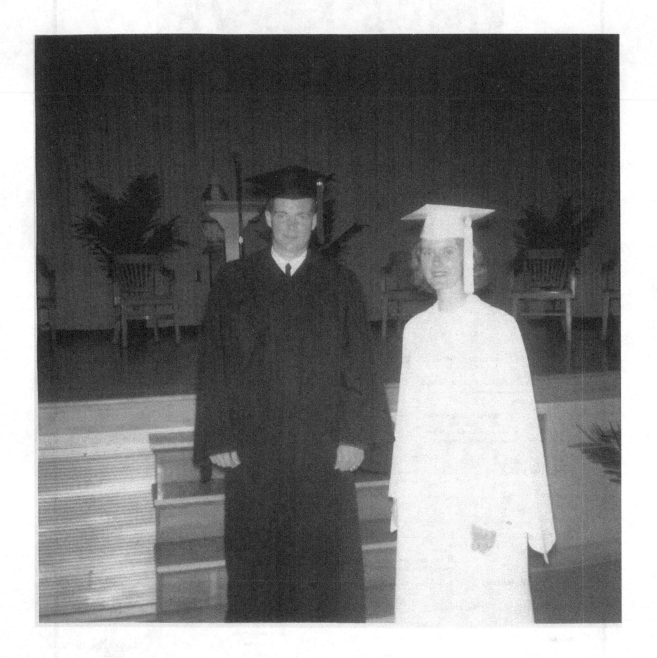

THE 'VOLUNTEER'

Dear Folks,

Talked to NROTC people here. If I pass my physical I can go into the contract program and thereby be eligible to go into the regular program after I pass a test in December.

Advantages of NROTC over AFROTC

1) terminate anytime before my junior year.

2) already in the so-called "advanced" program, that is, if I want to go on to get a commission there is no question that I'll be able to get it.

3) summer cruise — not until summer after junior year.

4) eligible in two ways for *regular navy program

1) through passing test

2) through appointment by base commander. O.S.U.

*regular program pays everything plus $50 a month. (that is, books, tuition etc.)

Please fill out forms and send them back as soon as possible.

Started checking account at Ohio National, picked up check # 100.00 at Bursar's Office and deposited it with $150.00 bank money order. Will buy theatre and activities ticket tomorrow. Will have to wait to get schedule adjusted until I find out if I can get in NROTC. Meanwhile, I'll drop my Spanish.

I've got enough money for quite a~~ awhile — meanwhile I'm being given quite a rush-around. Had lunch at ΣN, now heading to TKE for supper.

This is supposed to be just a <u>short</u> note to ask you to hurry the forms back so I guess I'd better close now.

Love

Ron

P.S. Take care, be good, and let me know how everything is on your end of the line.

CONTRACT FOR CONTRACT STUDENT (NROTC)
NAVPERS 918 (Rev. 2–62)

CONTRACT STUDENT (NROTC) AGREEMENT between THE UNITED STATES OF AMERICA, Department of the Navy, and

RONALD   FRANK   DOYLE
(Type or print full name of Obligor)

This agreement is entered into between the United States of America, represented by the officer signing this agreement, and the above-named Obligor (with consent of parent or guardian, if under 21 years of age).

WHEREAS, Obligor, in consideration of the benefits which will accrue to him by reason of his membership in the Naval Reserve Officers Training Corps, agrees to enter upon and continue training therein as a Contract student until the completion of such training as may be prescribed leading to an appointment as a Reserve officer of the United States Navy or as a Reserve officer of the United States Marine Corps, and to accept such appointment, if offered; and

WHEREAS, Obligor agrees to remain unmarried until commissioned; and

WHEREAS, Obligor understands that; in view of this agreement, he will be deferred from induction for service under the Universal Military Training and Service Act, as amended, until after completion or termination of the course of instruction, and, thereafter, so long as he continues in a reserve status upon being commissioned. Notwithstanding the foregoing, the Obligor understands that he is required to comply with all requirements of law as they pertain to registration for selective service.

WHEREAS, Obligor understands that the Chief of Naval Personnel may release him from his obligations under this agreement and separate him from the training program at any time that, in the opinion of the Chief of Naval Personnel, the best interests of the Naval Service require such action.

NOW, THEREFORE, the Parties hereto do hereby agree as follows:

TERM OF SERVICE. Obligor is hereby obligated to serve for the full period of active duty and inactive duty herein specified as follows:

1. The Obligor understands that, if he completes the prescribed training and is appointed to commissioned grade in the Navy or Marine Corps, he must serve on active duty for not less than three years after receipt of commission.
2. The Obligor agrees to retain a commission until the sixth anniversary of receipt of original commission in the United States Naval Service.
3. Upon completion of active duty in the Naval Service, Obligor will be placed in the Ready Reserve if eligible therefor. Service in the Ready Reserve will be for a period which when added to his active duty will total five years. Upon completion of this five years of satisfactory service on active duty and in the Ready Reserve he will be eligible for transfer to the Standby Reserve and if he applies he will be transferred to the Standby Reserve for any remaining portion of his service obligation.
4. The Obligor understands that the provisions of law require satisfactory participation in the Ready Reserve unless relieved of such participation by competent authority. Such participation may be satisfied annually by not less than 48 drills and not more than 17 days active duty for training or an alternative of 30 days active duty for training or other appropriate Reserve training as may be authorized. Failure to perform prescribed training in any year may subject him to involuntary call to active duty for not more than 45 days.
5. The Obligor understands that, if his obligated period of active duty under this agreement expires in time of war or national emergency proclaimed by the President, he may be involuntarily retained on active duty beyond such obligated period.

IN WITNESS WHEREOF, the Parties hereto have executed this agreement.

_____   Ronald Frank Doyle
(Witness to signature of Obligor)   *(Signature in full of Obligor)*

I, _____, parent/legal guardian of _____ _____, whose signature appears on the foregoing contractual agreement, do hereby consent to his entering into such contractual agreement.

_____   _____
(Date)   *(Parent/Legal Guardian)*

DO NOT WRITE BELOW THIS LINE

Subscribed to this   UNITED STATES OF AMERICA
          By direction of Secretary of the Navy

_____ day of

_____, 19

_____
Professor of Naval Science

CONTRACT NROTC PROGRAM REQUIREMENT INFORMATION

While in college a Contract NROTC student may take any course which leads to a baccalaureate or higher degree, except those which may be prohibited to NROTC students by the college or university.   This does not, however, entitle the student to any delay of active duty requirements after attaining the basic requirements for commissioning should he be pursuing any course that would normally require additional graduate work prior to becoming qualified for his profession.   NROTC students are required to take, in addition to the requirements of their major, 24 semester hours of Naval Science; they must complete satisfactorily by the end of their second year in the program one of the following:

a. Mathematics through trigonometry (in secondary school or college),
b. One semester OR quarter of college mathematics;

and they must achieve proficiency in written and oral expression in English, meeting the standards established by the college which they attend.   Students taking courses which do not require mathematics, but who must take mathematics to meet the requirements of the NROTC program, are advised that they may be confronted with scheduling difficulties and with an academic load that should only be attempted by outstanding students.   Physics is not required by the Navy for NROTC Contract students.   However, it is highly desirable if their academic schedule permits.

One summer cruise of approximately six weeks duration will be required.   This cruise is normally scheduled during the summer between the junior and senior years.

In order to permit the establishment of academic schedules, the screening and selection of Contract NROTC students must be completed in a very short time.   Certain final reviews cannot be completed in the time available.   Therefore, enrollment is authorized subject to the completion of a review of the report of physical examination in the Bureau of Medicine and Surgery, and review of the application file in the Bureau of Naval Personnel, which may not be accomplished until the spring of the first academic year.   A student found not qualified for enrollment in the program will be advised at the earliest practical time.   But he may, if he so desires, be retained in the program until the end of the current academic year in order that there will be no loss of academic credit.   If so retained he will be dropped from the program effective the last day of the academic year.

Each Contract NROTC student, if in all respects qualified, is required to accept a Reserve Commission in the United States Navy or Marine Corps and to serve on active duty for a period of three years.   All Contract NROTC students receiving commissions are required to retain their commissions for a total period of six years, unless sooner released by the Secretary of the Navy.

1 JUN 65

DEAR RON,

WELL, HOW IS IT GOING? YOU SHOULD BE GETTING OUT OF SCHOOL ABOUT NOW. I HOPE YOU GET THIS LETTER BEFORE YOU CUT OUT FOR HOME.

ANOTHER MONTH SHOT. ONLY $7\frac{1}{2}$ MORE TO GO. REALLY NOT TOO MUCH HAPPENING OVER HERE. I'M STILL PRETTY BUSY, BUT THE SAME OLD STUFF GETS OLD.

I FINALLY BOUGHT MY STEREO. I'VE GOT ALL THE COMPONENTS I NEED FOR AWHILE. BEFORE I GO HOME I'LL GET A RECORD CHANGER-TURNTABLE. THAT SHOULD FINISH THE SET OFF. THIS GIVES ME SOMETHING TO WORK ON AFTER DUTY HOURS.

HOW WAS YOUR SEMESTER? DID YOU GET OUT ANY? WHAT SUBJECTS DID YOU TAKE? THE NEXT TIME YOU MAKE IT DOWN TO THE HEIDELBURG - TIP A FEW FOR ME.

I'M MANAGING TO SPEND QUITE A BIT OF MONEY OVER HERE. IT'S NOT HARD AT ALL. EVENTUALLY, I HOPE TO START SAVING SOME. FINANCE STILL HAS MY ALLOTMENT SCREWED UP. RIGHT NOT I HAVE BEEN OVER PAID $400.00 WHICH THEY'LL TAKE OUT ONE OF THESE DAYS.

OH WELL, IT'S ALL PART OF THE HARDSHIP TOUR. TAKE IT EASY & MAKE SOME MONEY THIS SUMMER

Z-47

E. I. du Pont de Nemours & Company
INCORPORATED
P. O. Box 1217
PARKERSBURG, W. VA. 26181

PLASTICS DEPARTMENT

September 23, 1965

Mr. Ronald F. Doyle
1004 - 44th Street
Vienna, West Virginia

Dear Ron:

We hope that you gained some profitable experience at Washington Works during the past summer. We certainly enjoyed having you with us.

Your contribution to the plant was appreciated and helped us satisfy our customer demands during a period of peak production. We trust that the experience and training you received will be beneficial in your future pursuits. One of the specific benefits, which we hope you have acquired, is a respect for safety and its importance in all of your activities.

Thank you, again, and good luck!

Sincerely,

R. T. MURRILL
Works Manager

cws

Plate A-16a: OSU Work-Study

STUDENT COPY

THE OHIO STATE UNIVERSITY
NOTICE OF TRANSFER

Today's Date 2-9-67

Full Legal Name __DOYLE__ __RONALD__ __FRANK__   Soc. Sec. # __235-70-8053__
　　　　　　　　　　Last　　First　　Middle or Maiden

Permanent Address __1004 44TH ST__ __VIENNA W. VA.__
　　　　　　　　Number and Street　　　　　　City and State　　　　　Zip Code

Mailing Address __47 E 17TH AVE__ __COLUMBUS__ Columbus Telephone __—__
　　　　　　　Number and Street　　　　City and State

Marital Status:　　　Single ✓　Married ☐　　　Birth Date __MAY 2, 1946__

Transfer (Admission) Request From __Com__ _____ To __art__
　　　　　　　　　　　　　College, School, Combination Curriculum　　　　College, School, Combination Curriculum
　　　　　　　　　　　　　　　　　　　　(If in Graduate School, print only "GRAD" above)

Proposed Major or Field of Specialization __GEOGRAPHY__

COLLEGES OR UNIVERSITIES ATTENDED AND DEGREES HELD:

College or University	Dates Attended	Degree Conferred and Date
College or University	Dates Attended	Degree Conferred and Date
College or University	Dates Attended	Degree Conferred and Date

To Be Filled Out by All Applicants Except Those Applying to the Graduate School

Reason for transfer (Optional) _____

Total OSU Credit Hours (Incl. present qtr.) __139__   Last Attended OSU __WINTER__ _____ Quarter, 19 67
Total Number of Quarters attended (from last grade report) __7__　　　(Include Current Quarter)
Were you ever dismissed from OSU? __NO__ If "YES," was dismissal waived? __—__
When? __—__ _____ Name of college? __—__

Check the campus you will attend:　　　✓ Columbus　☐ Lima　☐ Mansfield
☐ Marion　☐ Newark　☐ Wright-Patterson AFB　☐ Other _____

List the courses on your schedule for the present quarter:

ENGLISH 505	GERMAN 401
POLI SCI 507	
CHINESE 511	

Present OSU Class Rank ☐1 ☐2 ✓3 ☐4
OSU Acc. Pt. Hr. Ratio __3.099__
Qtr. & Yr. First Admitted to OSU: __FALL 1964__
OSU Degree to be Conferred __SPRING 1968__
　　　　　　　　　　　　　　Qtr./Yr.

ADMISSIONS OFFICE USE ONLY:　　　CPHR _____ TOTAL HOURS _____ Certificate# _____

Transfer From __Com__ To __Art__ Grad. Dept. _____ Effective __Spr__ Quarter, 19 67
　　　　Include Location　　Include Location

Provisional For _____
Conditions _____

CHANGE STATUS　FROM: Regular _____ , Special _____ , Transnt. _____ , Irreg. _____
　　　　　　　　　TO: Regular _____ , Special _____ , Transnt. _____ , Irreg. _____

✓ Transfer　☐ Readmission　Approved __Frishmore__ DATE __2-9-67__ BY __CJ__

SEE REVERSE SIDE FOR CONDITIONS OF TRANSFER

Plate A-16b: OSU Work-Study

THE OHIO STATE UNIVERSITY
STUDENT FINANCIAL AIDS
154 W. 12th Avenue
Columbus, Ohio 43210

TO: RONALD DOYLE   JUN 13 1967

SUBJECT: WORK AUTHORIZATION

You (are) not eligible for a CW-SP job. Your 1967-68 NEED BALANCE is $ _111400_

You may work long enough to make up your NEED BALANCE, then you must leave your CW-SP job.

~~Your NEED BALANCE is too small to permit you to~~ ~~quarter~~
~~must quit your CW-SP job on~~ ~~work~~ ~~quarter~~
19 ~~If you submit a report of your resources during the period you did not have a CW-SP~~
~~job and if our evaluation at that time establishes a significant NEED BALANCE.~~

NOTE: Let Us Compute Your Need Balance Which Establishes Your Eligibility For A CW-SP Job.

        DO NOT TRY TO COMPUTE YOUR NEED BALANCE YOURSELF.

Keep a running total on the NEED BALANCE Record Form below, of all NET earnings received
from ALL sources after 15 June 1967. Add to this running total all NEW resources. This
consists of any resources not reported on the application and financial statements (blue
forms) you recently submitted. Here are examples of NEW resources: (1) parents give you
more than shown on "blue forms", (2) you receive a new scholarship, loan, etc., or the
amount was changed or, (3) your spouse earns more or less than estimated on the "blue form".
When your running total comes within $150.00 of your NEED BALANCE, telephone (293-7363)
and talk personally to Mr. Bobo. DO NOT DELAY DISCUSSION.

                                     Carl E. Bobo, Jr.
                                     Manager College Work-Study Program

- -

                          NEED BALANCE RECORD FORM

                Record: Running Total

                (1) ALL NET EARNINGS

                (2) ALL NEW RESOURCES

1967-68 NEED BALANCE $ _1114 00_

  Reported on "blue forms".
 *Parents Contribution $ _2080 00_
 *Spouse's Earnings
 *Scholarship Ken Univ. $ _250 00_
 *Loan $
 *Grant $
 *Other

* If there is any change in the above, telephone
  Mr. Bobo, 293-7363, as soon as possible.

OSU TRANSCRIPTS 1964-68

OFFICE OF THE REGISTRAR — THE OHIO STATE UNIVERSITY, COLUMBUS, OHIO

Name: DOYLE, RONALD FRANK
Address: Vienna, West Virginia

Admission Information: Parkersburg, West Virginia, Catholic High School, May 1961

AUTUMN QTR 1964

Title of Course	Department	Course Number	Credit Hours	Grade	Points
INTRO W EUROP LIT	COMP LIT	401	3	A	12
COMPOSITION & RDG	ENGLISH	416	3	B	9
W WORLD MOD TIMES	HISTORY	421	5	A	20
ALGEBRA & TRIG	MATH	439	5	B	15
ORIENTATION	SRV ARTS	401	0		
HYGIENE	HLTH EDU	400	1	B	3
REQUIRED	PHYS ED	401	1	R	3
			18	3.444	62

18   3.444   62

WINTER QTR 1965

INTRO W EUROP LIT	COMP LIT	402	3	A	12
COMPOSITION & RDG	ENGLISH	417	3	B	9
W 19TH CENTURY	HISTORY	422	5	A	20
CALC ANALYT GEOM	MATH	440	5	C	10
REQUIRED	PHYS ED	402	1	B	3
			17	3.176	54

35   3.314   116

SPRING 1965

INTRO W EUROP LIT	COMP LIT	403	3	B	9
COMPOSITION & RDG	ENGLISH	418	3	C	6
ELEMENTARY FRENCH	FRENCH	401	5	A	20
W WLD 20TH CENTURY	HISTORY	423	5	A	20
REQUIRED	PHYS ED	403	1	B	3
			17	3.411	58

52   3.346   174

TRANSFERRED to Commerce September 1965.

AUTUMN 1965

PRINS OF BIOLOGY	BIOLOGY	402	5	B	15
ELEMENTARY FRENCH	FRENCH	402	5	C	15
INTRODUCTION	GEOG	401	5	A	20
INTRO TO THEATRE	SPEECH	430	3	B	9
			18	3.277	59

70   3.328   233

WINTER 1966

GENERAL BOTANY	BOTANY	403	5	A	20
CLASS CIVIL GREECE	CL LANG	524	3	A	12
PRINCIPLES OF ECON	ECON	501	5	A	20
ECONOMIC GEOGRAPHY	GEOG	403	5	C	10
			18	3.444	62

88   3.352   295

COLLEGE OF COMMERCE — ARTS AND SCIENCES

Entered Sept 22...   Graduated...   Degree...

Name: DOYLE, RONALD FRANK
Date of Birth: May 2, 1946
Place of Birth: LIVINGSTON, NEW JERSEY

SPRING 1965

Title of Course	Department	Course Number	Credit Hours	Grade	Pts.
INTRODUCTION	ACCTING	501	5	B	1
PRINCIPLES OF ECON	ECON	502	5	B	2
CALC & ANALYT GEOM	MATH	441	5	D	3
			15	2.333	

103   3.203   330

AUTUMN QUARTER 1966

INTRODUCTION	ACCTING	502	5	C	1
CONTRACT RELATNSHP	BUS ORG	621	4	B	1
ELEM ECON STAT	ECON	542	4	C	1
MONEY AND BANKING	ECON	623			
			18	2.500	4

121   3.099   375

WINTER QUARTER 1967

ELEM CHINESE THOT	CHINESE	571	3	A	1
INFORMATIVE WRITNG	ENGLISH	505	5	B	1
ELEMENTARY GERMAN	GERMAN	401	5	A	2
FUNDAMENTLS GOVT	POLIT SC	507	5	B	1
			18	3.444	c

139   3.143   437

TRANSFERRED to Arts March 1967

SPRING QUARTER 1967

LOCALIZATN MFG IND	GEOG	603	3	C	
INTRODUCTION	GEOLOGY	416	5	C	
ELEMENTARY GERMAN	GERMAN	402	5	A	
PHIL BASES W CULTR	PHILOS	520	5	B	
			18	2.833	

157   3.108   488

SUMMER QUARTER 1967

FUNDAMENTALS	SOCIOL	507	5	A	2
			5	4.000	

162   3.135   508

COURSE NUMBERING SYSTEM CHANGED EFFECTIVE SEPTEMBER 1967

AUTUMN QUARTER 1967

CLIMATOLOGY	GEOG	520	4	B
POLITICAL GEOG	GEOG	560	3	A
URBAN GEOGRAPHY	GEOG	650	3	A
INTERMEDIATE	GERMAN	103	5	C

3.114   174   542   174   2.833 — 12
177   554   177   15

MARKING SYSTEM

July 1922:
A—Excellent
B—Good
C—Average
D—Poor
E—Failed
EM—Abs—Failed absent
Ex—Examination Credit
I—Incomplete
K—Transferred credit

August 1955:
F—Failure absent (E abs)
I—Incomplete
N—None required
P—Progress
R—Final report will be reported at end of sequence

October 1961:
R—Registered as Audit "R—Final Mark" and "U—Audit" are cancelled

February 1961:
A—Highest Quality
B—Second Quality
C—Third Quality
D—Lowest Quality

September 1963:
H—Honors (Medicine only)
S—satisfactory (Grad and Medicine)

Courses numbered 600 or above carry no credit toward a degree in the Graduate...

Admission Authorization '68

return to file

March 21, 1968

Mr. Ronald F. Doyle
118 West 10th Avenue
Columbus, Ohio   43201

Dear Mr. Doyle:

I am happy to inform you that you have been awarded a teaching assistantship for the 1968-69 academic year. The stipend is $2,250 for three quarters. All tuition fees will be waived, both in-state and out-of-state. Duties will consist of meeting two or less weekly discussion sections for a total not to exceed four contact hours. For subsequent years there are excellent possibilities of increased financial support. Students with the Master's degree are eligible , after one year in the Department, for Teaching Associateships with a three-quarter stipend of $3,600. Research assistantships are also available to second-year students who are participating in faculty research projects.

We have a young and vigorous faculty at Ohio State, currently engaged in a variety of research projects as well as in new and imaginative approaches to their teaching. As you know we feel we are particularly strong in political geography with three faculty members specializing in that topic.

You have until April 15 to formally accept or reject your award but we would, of course, appreciate being notified as soon as possible after you have made your decision. If you have any questions, don't hesitate to call collect, 293-2514 (Area Code 614). We hope you decide to join us, and are looking forward to hearing from you.

Sincerely,

Edward J. Taaffe
Chairman
Department of Geography

EJT/jlk

THE VIETNAM ERA
Troubled Times...

HARDING HOSPITAL
DIAGNOSIS:
BRAIN DISORDER
1968

UNAFFECTED   AFFECTED

HYDROCLEANING

Heist

SUMMERS '69, '70

AT MOBAY
AND OTHER OHIO VALLEY PLANTS

EXECUTIVE ASSISTANT
ROUTE PLANNING DEPARTMENT
JUNE-DECEMBER 1971

RONALD F. DOYLE   (614) 468-9740

CCS
CONSUMER
COMMUNICATION
SERVICES CORPORATION

1140 CHESAPEAKE AVENUE • COLUMBUS, OHIO 43212

BACHELOR
OF
ARTS
1969

MASTER OF ARTS
1971

THE STUDENT UNION

DISTURBANCES AT O.S.U. 1970

THE GRADUATE SCHOOL
OHIO STATE UNIVERSITY
GEOGRAPHY DEPARTMENT
GRADUATE TEACHING ASSISTANT
SEPTEMBER 1969-JUNE 1971

IMPAIRED AND IMPERILED
MY EARLY CAREER YEARS
1968-1973

CUYAHOGA COMMUNITY COLLEGE
METRO CAMPUS, CLEVELAND, OHIO
VISITING LECTURER (GEOGRAPHY)
JANUARY-JUNE 1972

In The Heart
Of The Recently
Quieted Cleveland
Black Ghetto

Ronald Frank Doyle
SELECTIVE SERVICE NO. 16 20 46 353
May 2 1946 Livingston N. J.
Blue Brown 5 ft 10 in 135

PROGRESSIVE
SELECTIVE SERVICE
CLASSIFICATIONS:
2-S / 1-A / 1-Y / 4-F

EXPLORING
NORTH
AMERICA

1969,1970,1972

CHANGING JOBS:
(LATE 1972 & 1973)

DEPT STORE STOCKPERSON

A CARIBBEAN ADVENTURE

ECON. DEV. PLANNER

AIRPORT LIMO DRIVER

CHAPTER THREE

IMPAIRED & IMPERILED

Scary Adventures of My Early Work Career
(1968-1973): 9% OF MY LIFE BEFORE AGE 62
[May 1968 to November 1973: 6 years, 7 months]

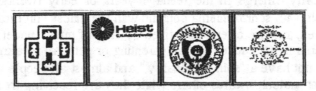

THE PRELUDE: PERSONAL HISTORY 1968-1973
WEATHERING "THE PERFECT STORM" OF MY YOUNG LIFE

In the spring of 1968, my parents say, I suddenly began talking and acting alarmingly bizarrely. Unsure as to what to do, my parents consulted with a local doctor-friend who advised them to have me hospitalized and treated at a Columbus area psychiatric hospital. There, at Harding Hospital, I was diagnosed with paranoid schizophrenia and treated with a number of anti-psychotic drugs which had mental and physical side effects of their own. Finally released after a couple of months and told to "Avoid stress!" I returned to living on the OSU campus on medication and mentally impaired compared to what I was before the schizophrenic attacks and the primitive drug therapy that was available then.

After working briefly as an order picker at a local warehouse, I returned to studies at OSU with the help of a male nurse from Harding Hospital named Brent Demlow and completed requirements for my B.A. degree in June 1969. I then attended graduate school where I was a teaching assistant during the University's time of troubles (the civil disturbance, riots, and school closing in the spring of 1970). In June of 1971 I received my M.A. in geography. During the preceding summers I worked for C.H. Heist Corporation doing industrial hydrocleaning.

Following this period I went into the job market still impaired from schizophrenia and the drug therapy. For a couple of years (1971-1973) I went from job to job trying to find something I could do successfully for more than a couple of months at a time. In too rapid succession I was:

- a planner at an independent postal service (Columbus, OH);
- a visiting lecturer at a community college in the heart of the recently quieted Cleveland black ghetto;
- a cab driver (Parkersburg, WV);
- a light truck driver (Parkersburg to Cleveland route);
- a department store warehouseman (Vienna, WV);
- a water jet operator-pumpman (Ponce, PR);
- a government planner (Parkersburg, WV); and,
- an airport limousine driver (Parkersburg, WV).

Schizophrenia

What is schizophrenia?

Schizophrenia is a serious and challenging medical illness, an illness that affects well over 2 million American adults, which is about 1 percent of the population age 18 and older. Although it is often feared and misunderstood, schizophrenia is a treatable medical condition.

Schizophrenia often interferes with a person's ability to think clearly, to distinguish reality from fantasy, to manage emotions, make decisions, and relate to others. The first signs of schizophrenia typically emerge in the teenage years or early twenties, often later for females. Most people with schizophrenia contend with the illness chronically or episodically throughout their lives, and are often stigmatized by lack of public understanding about the disease. Schizophrenia is not caused by bad parenting or personal weakness. A person with schizophrenia does not have a "split personality," and almost all people with schizophrenia are not dangerous or violent towards others while they are receiving treatment. The World Health Organization has identified schizophrenia as one of the ten most debilitating diseases affecting human beings.

What are the symptoms of schizophrenia?

No one symptom positively identifies schizophrenia. All of the symptoms of this illness can also be found in other mental illnesses. For example, psychotic symptoms may be caused by the use of illicit drugs, may be present in individuals with Alzheimer's disease, or may be characteristics of a manic episode in bipolar disorder. However, when a doctor observes the symptoms of schizophrenia and carefully assesses the history and the course of the illness over six months, he or she can almost always make a correct diagnosis.

As with any other psychiatric diagnosis, it is important to have a good medical work-up to be sure the diagnosis is correct. Drug use can mimic the symptoms of schizophrenia and may also trigger vulnerability in individuals at risk. Other medical concerns also need to be ruled out before a correct diagnosis can be made.

How is schizophrenia treated?

While there is no cure for schizophrenia, it is a treatable and manageable illness. However, people sometimes stop treatment because of medication side effects, the lack of insight noted above, disorganized thinking, or because they feel the medication is no longer working. People with schizophrenia who stop taking prescribed medication are at risk of relapse into an acute psychotic episode. It's important to realize that the needs of the person with schizophrenia may change over time. Medication: The primary medications for schizophrenia are called antipsychotics. Antipsychotics help relieve the positive symptoms of schizophrenia by helping to correct an imbalance in the chemicals that enable brain cells to communicate with each other. As with drug treatments for other physical illnesses, many patients with severe mental illnesses may need to try several different antipsychotic medications before they find the one, or the combination of medications, that works best for them.

(http://www.namimi.org/schizophrenia?gclid=CLyejbLk8agCFU5qKgoda2i Gw, May 18, 2011)

EFFECTS OF ANTI-PSYCHOTIC MEDICATIONS PRESCRIBED:

Chlorpromazine
THORAZINE

Fluphenazine
PROLIXIN

Thioridazine
MELLARIL

Haloperidol
HALDOL

Triflouperazine
STELAZINE

Thiothixene
NAVANE

SPECIAL MENTAL AND PHYSICAL SIDE EFFECTS

MENTAL EFFECTS: Confusion, Delirium, Short-term Memory Problems, Disorientation, and Impaired Attention.

PHYSICAL EFFECTS: Dry Mouth, Constipation, Difficulty Urinating, Blurred Vision, Decreased Sweating With Increased Body Temperature, Sexual Dysfunction, and Worsening of Glaucoma.

NOTE: All of these drugs are effective for treating mental illnesses called psychoses, including schizophrenia. They should not be used to treat anxiety; to sedate...or control restless behavior or other problems of non-psychotic people. These anti-psychotics can cause serious side-effects, including...the "jitters", and weakness and muscle fatigue.

Source: WORST PILLS BEST PILLS: THE OLDER ADULT'S GUIDE TO AVOIDING DRUG-INDUCED DEATH OR ILLNESS by Wolfe, Fugate, Holstrand, Kamimoto and Public Citizen Health Research Group.

Typically, after finally securing a job I would work hard at it. But, due to mental confusion and other disabilities, I'd soon fail to perform well. I would then leave the job rather than be fired (or, sometimes I was fired) and search for a new job repeating the process again. Needless to say this was a very unhappy time in my life with few uplifting occurrences.

In addition, from 1968 until January 1972, I was eligible for the military draft. While down-classified (I-Y) because of my schizophrenia, in the event of 'war or national emergency' I would be taken. This was not an inconsiderable worry to me as schizophrenia and guns never did mix well and I was having considerable difficulty handling the stress of normal civilian living, let alone war! However, in January 1972 I was reclassified 4-F (unfit for military service). This was like taking the top off a pressure cooker! Gradually afterward my health improved.

While I remember my time with each employer of the period, my time with one employer, C.H. Heist Corporation, is remembered more favorably than my times with the others as my schizophrenia seemed to clear briefly to allow me to work and show my true character with them, evidencing enough "piss and vinegar" to do a difficult job somewhat well and earning me "virtue" or "karma" I did not have before my employment with them.

What follows covers three times of employment: summer 1969; summer 1970; and January to March 1973. The dangers that the job presented were not the fault of C.H. Heist Corp. But rather were presented by the entire industry and by the times. I remain grateful to C.H. Heist for employing me again and again when few others, some rightly so, would readily have me. I am respectful of the many brave workers of the industrial hydrocleaning industry past and present in the chemical plants of the world.

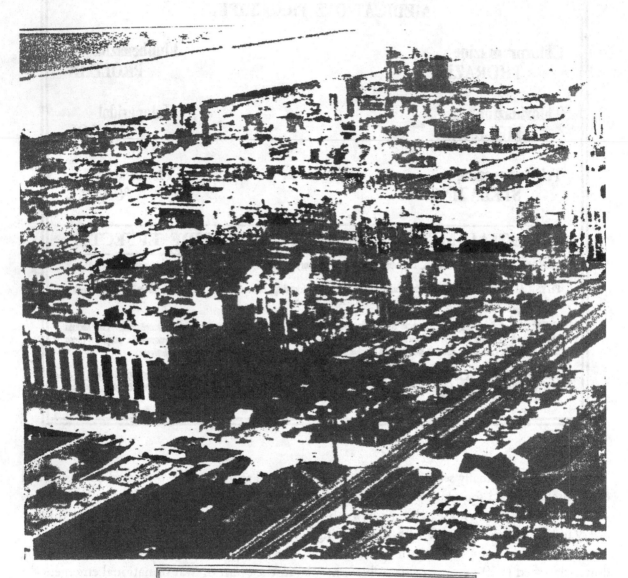

MOBAY Chemical, New Martinsville, WV in the late 1960s

PART I

THE WORK

Excerpt 1

June to September 1969: Mobay Chemical and Other Mid-Ohio Valley Plants

MOBAY: MY SUMMER JOB 1969

My parents and I had decided that I would go on to graduate school in late 1969 (rather than to attempt a career job was harder or try to get a full-time job with a bachelor's degree in geography which would be still harder.) Meanwhile my father arranged a job for me with C.H. Heist Corporation as a summer employee.

The work was physically hard and dirty, somewhat dangerous, but mentally non-taxing. Since there were few people who wanted to do this kind of work, the pay for an unskilled young man was relatively high—allowing me to squirrel monies away for the next school year's expenses. We worked in the plants of the Mid-Ohio Valley and beyond, from Ravenswood (then Kaiser Aluminum) to Pittsburgh (The Edgar J. Thompson Works). But mostly I was assigned to MOBAY, a large facility in New Martinsville, WV which made a wide variety of chemical products for private industry and the government, including phosgene, a nerve gas, and tear gas.

> **HISTORICAL NOTE:** As I understood it, during the Cold War both Congress and the President agreed on the necessity of the MAD program—the manufacture and stockpiling of poisonous gas and biochemical agents of mass destruction leading to a 'balance of terror with the Soviet Union which was making its own stockpiles. In theory this would keep the peace at least between the superpowers themselves, since war between the superpowers *directly* would be 'too horrible.' Thus, the work contributed to peace and I had no moral hang-ups about it. This program was known as the MAD program (Mutual Assured Destruction).

Most often, while there, I worked in the phosgene/tear gas area. MOBAY personnel seldom were engaged in the dirty and dangerous work themselves. They brought in outside contractors from all over the U.S. (like C.H. Heist) to do that and paid them well—also heading off unionization attempts of their own highly skilled work force.

The managers and scientists there then wore brown uniforms (coveralls) and the mechanical people gray coveralls. For reference we called them the 'brown shirts' and the 'gray shirts'

BILL PERFORMS AN UNSCHEDULED DEMO . . .

Phosgene is a potently deadly nerve gas: tasteless, colorless, odorless, it penetrates through the pores of the skin. So, there is no defense against it—gas masks do nothing to protect. There was, however, an antidote that presumably was available in the plant hospital nearby on the plant grounds (also known as the plant 'campus').

Phosgene manufacture is largely an automatic process. But, in order to keep the gas made potently deadly, the interiors of the pipes of the process needed to be perfectly clean—no contaminants to weaken the blend. Consequently, every so often, a line would be shut down, all the pipes disassembled, and laid out for hydroblasting of the piping interiors. Before disassembly, I was told, air had been blown through the process pipes evacuating most of the phosgene in a specific piping system. Nevertheless, nerve gas pockets occasionally existed in the elbow joints, and in more complicated pipe pieces.

I was working in the phosgene facility but two days when Bill, my crew leader, after instructing me as to how dangerous this gas was, urged me to stand aside while he began hydroblasting a piece of pipe with an elbow in it . . .

Suddenly, he reared back, began to whirl and vomit profusely. The other two experienced team workers rushed toward him pushing him back away from the invisible cloud that had emerged from the pipe. Bill collapsed onto the concrete and passed out while the other two, now stricken too, retreated away. Finding my legs (they had frozen—I was temporarily petrified) I then rushed into the fray toward Bill. Somehow, seconds before, the wind slightly shifted and I was not touched by the cloud. I lifted up Bill's head and began rubbing it (not knowing what to do). Suddenly, Bill opened his eyes . . . By this time the other two had now recovered from their slight attacks and were glaring at me because Bill, just now conscious, was thanking me. A few eye-looks and a grin however straightened the matter out.

In twenty minutes, after Bill recovered his wind, and had rested, as was the custom with these hardhats, since Bill had been the one most seriously scared, he went back and finished the task. This is how I learned about the effects of phosgene—"a little goes a long way". I also learned one method of overcoming fear that worked for me many times in the future.

Industrial accidents not un common in Mid-Ohio Valley

By TOM HRACH
The Marietta Times

The fire that killed three people at Shell Chemical Co. on Friday was the latest of many industrial accidents in the Mid-Ohio Valley over the years.

With chemical and power plants lining both sides of the Ohio River, the potential for accidents is always there, say workers.

The accident that most people still remember happened on April 27, 1978, at the Pleasants Power Station in Willow Island, W.Va.

A scaffolding collapsed during construction of the one of the cooling towers, dropping workers to the concrete. In total, 51 construction workers were killed in the accident.

Other industrial fires, explosions and accidents:

► DEC. 9, 1992 at Elkem Metals on Ohio 7 in Marietta. Four workers are injured, two seriously, in an explosion.

► MAY 13, 1988 at American Cyanamid in, Willow Island, W.Va. James A. Robinson Jr., 33, of Parkersburg, a general supervisor at the plant, is killed in an explosion. Two others are hurt.

► APRIL 22, 1987 at Eveready Battery Co. Inc. on Ohio 7 in Marietta. Fire injured three firefighters and caused extensive damage to a major portion of the plant.

► MAY 19, 1983 at Elkem Metals. Three workers are killed and three others are injured in an explosion caused by sparks from a torch. Killed were Donald A. Mason, 60, of 213 Alden Ave., Marietta; Rawleigh Jerry Keller, 35, of Walker, W.Va.;

and James Webb, 32, of Fleming.

► JUNE 17, 1985 at Energy Unlimited in Devola. One was killed and two others were injured when the three were cutting the tops off of empty anti-freeze drums with a blow torch that exploded. Killed was Douglas Clark, 22, of Caldwell.

► MARCH 16, 1981 at Ohio Power's Muskingum River plant near Beverly. Five workers are injured, two seriously, when a tank exploded.

► APRIL 17, 1975 at Shell Chemical in Belpre. An 18-year-old worker on his first day on the job was killed by a blast from a high-pressure water hose as he cleaned industrial equipment. Killed was Donald Henderson of Williamstown.

► JAN. 30, 1969 at Union Carbide Plastics on Ohio 7 in Marietta. Twelve were injured in an explosion.

TWO CUBAN SOLDIERS . . .

Later in the summer, since we worked on call irregular hours, I had been off a couple of days. When I was called back to work at MOBAY Bill told me all work had ceased several hours last Saturday because of a bomb threat. (A bomb properly placed and detonated in that place would have resulted in multiple explosions—taking most of New Martinsville with it depending on the winds.) Bill said the grapevine indicated two "touring" Cuban soldiers were responsible for telephoning in the threat. It was a tense time as evacuation was senseless. (It really was impossible to get all those hundreds of workers out of the plant to a safe distance in a reasonable amount of time.) The 'campus' was carefully searched by plant squads. No bomb was found. Work resumed.

(The incident could obviously be repeated anytime—and the next time the bomb could be real.)

HAVE FAITH BUT WORK RELIGIOUSLY—THE EXPLOSIVE VAT

One day in August our job was to clean out a vat that had chemically frozen over (hardened). Only one problem: a spark could cause the solidified material to ignite and explode. We used wooden chisels, a rubber mallet, and a small pneumatic jack hammer with its own fitted wooden chisel. One of the 'brown shirts' was with us every moment of the time—talking us on gently . . . We took frequent breaks, worked slowly and carefully. After a few days (rotating teams in shifts) the vat was clean. *We had hoped for the best but had a method.* I also grew some from that experience.

A HELP TO 'POOR' TOM—BUT, NEVER AGAIN, UNLESS REQUIRED

Tom was one of our workers with whom nobody would work. He was a little 'slow' but good spirited. Bill, our crew leader, asked for someone to work with Tom. None of the experienced people made a move. So, I volunteered. (After all, I was a little 'slow' now too). Bill hesitated, explaining . . . I still said OK. Bill, still needing someone, reluctantly OK'd my going to him.

Tom was cleaning out the tank in a tank truck parked toward the rear of the MOBAY plant. Because the truck's tank had contained fluids which if inhaled could induce "pneumonia" and still had a few inches of the stuff on the tank floor and in a coating on the tank walls, we wore our gas masks into the tank along with the usual rubberized suits and gloves. Tom helped me though the tank top of the tank truck. I descended to the tank floor. A light was handed in and I hung it on the air hose to my gas mask. "OK," I signaled. But Tom then thoughtlessly turned on the water full blast.

The tank floor was slippery. Immediately I lost my footing as the water pressure pinned me to the back wall. The light smashed out. Somehow the air hose did not snap however and I hung there precariously hi the darkness. About 15 minutes later, Tom looked down into the tank. "Oh," he said.

I came up through the tank top after Tom turned the water off. I peered into his face—but noticed no malice, just "no brains." I just asked him to turn the water back on a little less forcefully, careful to explain why. Then, as was our custom, since I was the one who had been most 'scared' I went back and finished the job. When I saw Bill again he just grinned and said, "That's why the guys like to let Tom work alone."

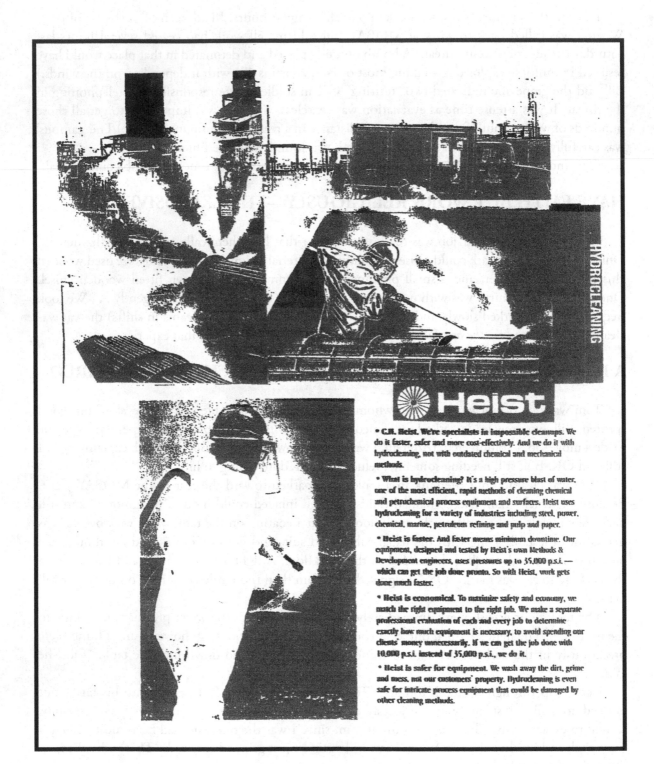

Excerpt 2

June and July 1970: (At MOBAY)

The marvels of modern chemistry continued to unfold to my young mind as I returned to MOBAY periodically to work during the summer of 1970.

A PANOPLY OF POISONOUS COLORS . . .

One morning I was called to MOBAY. Greathouse, one of the crew leaders, asked me to help him clean out a clogged sewer in a holding pond. As we arrived in the area of the pond in our filter masks. An early morning fog still enveloped the environs. As the sun's rays began to penetrate it as we worked what a picture emerged: the holding pond water was orange, the rocks along the shoreline were stained blue, and greenish clouds of chlorine gas shifted around above and among us as we cleaned the sewer pipe. I thought again about a 'conservative' bumper sticker on my neighbor's car: it read, "LET THE ENVIRONMENTALISTS FREEZE TO DEATH IN THE COLD AND THE DARK!" This was silly! There was a need for more environmental protection in 1970.

(That holding pond drained into the Ohio River.) Soon, the sewer was unclogged . . .

OTHER MEMORIES

Other memories of those days include but are not limited to:

- painting trestles at PPG seated 35 feet up on live rubber shielded high tension wires with bees swarming around being attracted to the paint,
- working with water and battery acid at Union Carbide's battery plant,
- helping a sandblaster at Kaiser Aluminum,
- and cleaning out the checkers under the blast furnace in the bowels of the Edgar J. Thompson steel mill with locomotives rumbling overhead.
- other scary experiences at Allied Chemical, Marbon, FMC, Electromet, the power plant and elsewhere.

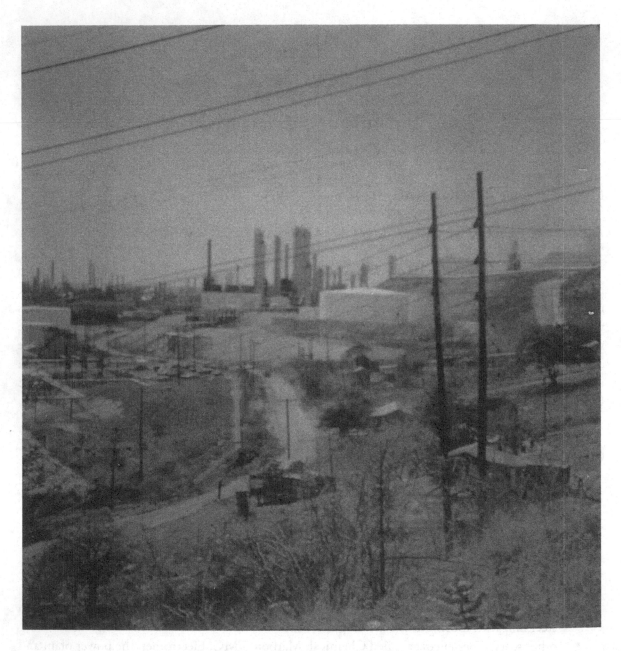

The industrial area around Ponce, PR, as it was in 1973

PART II

A CARIBBEAN ADVENTURE

Excerpt 3

January into March 1973: Puerto Rico

RETURN TO WORK AFTER FEELING ILL

Feeling better after Christmas and needing money to pay off a monetary debt I by then owed my father, I rejoined C.H. Heist doing the work I sincerely hated most, hydro-blasting.

Soon an opportunity came up to leave Parkersburg (it was winter and the ice formed by the water jet often froze on my hands) and work down in Puerto Rico. Without hesitation, I volunteered to go to the Ponce, PR site despite warnings from other workers who had been there of problems to North Americans working on the Island . . .

OUT OF THE ASHES RISES THE PHOENIX . . .

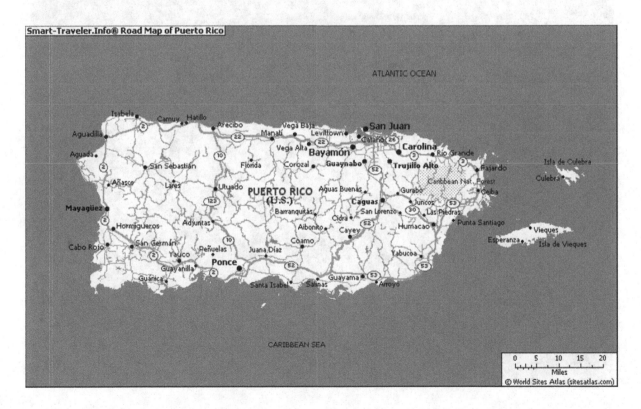

(from http://www.smart-traveler.info/map_of_pr.html, May 18, 2011)

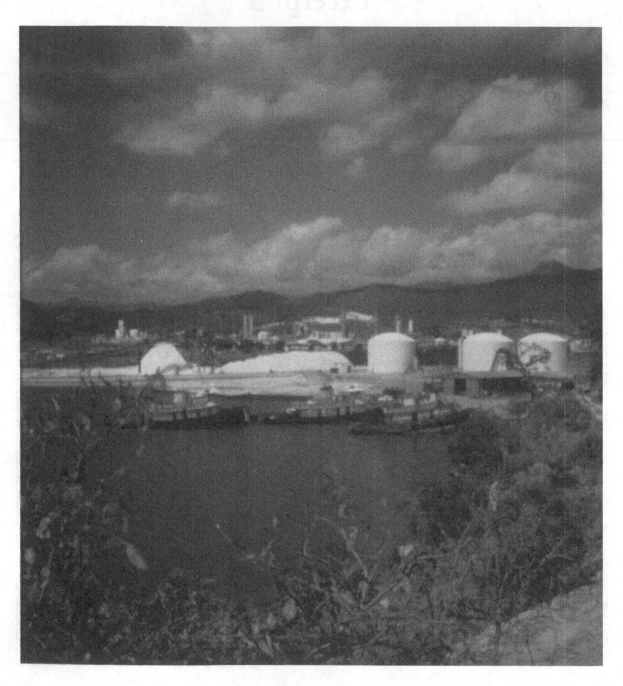

A port facility near Ponce

FORWARD AGAIN . . .

Tracy Jenkins explained to me on the plane down to Puerto Rico: we *Norde Americanos* would be somewhat less than welcome in Puerto Rico. As tourists it would have been almost A-OK. But, we were working there . . . and taking jobs that theoretically the local people could do. We were resented because our pay was higher (we got top wages accorded off-shore workers) and because unemployment throughout most of the island hovered in those days at about 20 percent. (Part of the reason we were being sent there was to help train local people to do our kind of work up to the quality standards set by the local (heavy) American manufacturing plants around Ponce.)

We would stay out of the bars . . . While no guns were permitted on the island (except police and military), those Puerto Ricans (a few among the many who might give us trouble) were renowned for their expertise with switchblade knives (and occasionally machetes out-of-doors).

The prohibition against guns also meant that throughout our stay we would be unarmed . . . That was no matter to me—I had never owned or used a gun—and I was the "type" to hesitate in pulling the trigger. (I was 90% *mouth* in those days, not fully able to protect myself yet.)

FROM SAN JUAN TO PONCE

Arriving in San Juan we quickly went over to the PRINAIR terminal for the flight to Ponce. PRINAIR, the local commuter airline, had a mixed reputation in those days. Many planes had been lost flying over those mountains into the interior. Being weighed and properly placed in the small plane also did not induce confidence. However, soon we were airborne as our 25 year old Latin pilot reassured us: "Don't worry, I've been well-trained . . ." But, we made it to Ponce in about an hour.

BEFORE THE SCREENING COMMITTEE

Once at the house the company had rented, the foreman, Rick, and John (the then current resident workers) began 'looking us over'. Tracy spoke first and after a few questions was easily accepted. Then I spoke. Silence followed for awhile—but I held my ground. Finally, a few questions were quietly put to me. My answers seemed to be intently listened to by the interviewers. Fortunately, (I was later told) I gave the right answers. (The wrong answers at this point would have quickly sent me back to the airport.)

'House rules' were introduced to us after we were both accepted. The foreman was 'in charge'. But, it worked this way: each resident had a vote and comment time to explain his vote. The foreman had his vote plus the number of votes of all the other residents summed together. On any divisive issues everyone got to vote and the foreman then decided.

Complaints against another were to be directed secretly to any third resident who then informed the one complained against matter-of-factly of the noted problem. Compliance was mandatory. (Complaints usually involved attitude problems or matters of personal hygiene.) This system worked like a 'charm'. Anger was never expressed and problems were quickly addressed and corrected in the crowded house. And an essential modest *espirit de corps* was built up quickly without much ado.

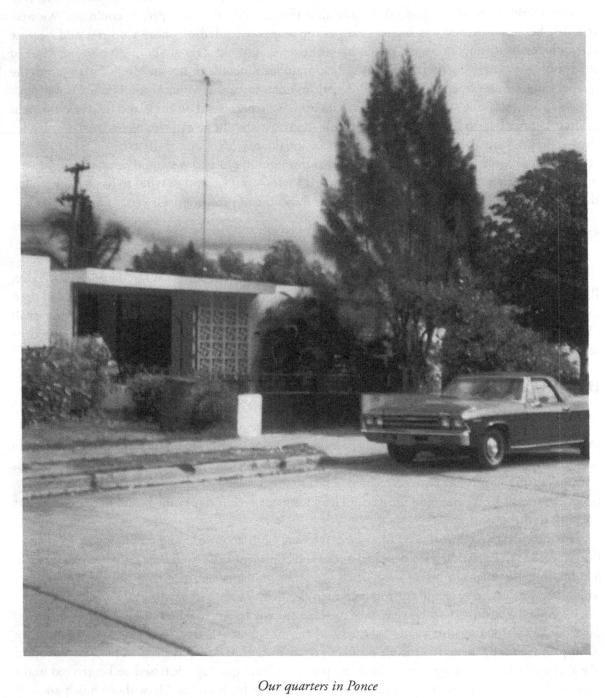

Our quarters in Ponce

JUAN STRIKES OUT AGAINST CAPITALISM.

The day before Tracy and I arrived, Juan, one of C. H. Heist Caribe Corporation's employees who had strong Marxist sentiments had attacked my immediate boss with a machete. While the other Puerto Ricans had stopped him before he reached the boss's body by tackling and subduing him, the incident had created some heartfelt bad impressions among the management.

But, things being the way they were on the island at that time (There was significant social friction between the left-wing (Marxist) political groups and the majority pro-U.S. citizenry), it was decided that it would be bad politics to report the incident to the police—the Marxists could argue that management was somehow mistreating Puerto Ricans and that Juan had struck 'a blow for freedom from Yankee imperialism' in self-defense—but management did fire him.

However, to repair feelings between ourselves (C.H. Heist Caribe Corporation) and the fired employee and his communist cell buddies and to maintain a favorable image of toleration and open-heartedness in the community at large, one of our foreman's assigned tasks was to occasionally visit him (Juan and other members of the cell were often distributing communist flyers to passing motorists downtown), be politely friendly, and take his literature "so that we can understand better".

So, occasionally the foreman took one or two of us along in the truck to visit Juan and his friends, and accept his literature.

The literature made good toilet paper when we ran low.

HISTORICAL NOTE: There had been an independence plebiscite on the island recently. The Puerto Rican independence movement had been overwhelmingly defeated at the election polls. (Continued commonwealth association drew the most votes.) Nevertheless, the Marxist and other independence-minded Puerto Ricans were still trying to line up another plebiscite. Currently, in 1973, the Marxists were most heavily trying to take over the labor movement (unions) on the island

---

INTO THE BARRIOS TO PICK UP OUR CREW

Our Puerto Rican workers tended to be from the poorest ranks of the Islanders, from among the 'barrio' people. Into the barrios we'd go every day with the company's battered green van, loading up our Puerto Rican crews (most of whom did not have cars) and taking them to the job sites. Always ready for trouble, we never had any.

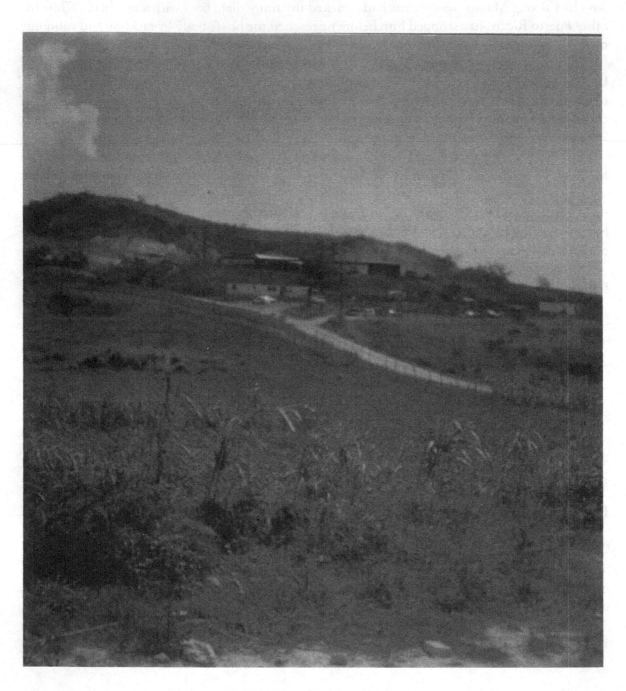

C. H. Heist base of local operations in 1973

> **HISTORICAL NOTE**: Government housing programs had just recently begun in the early 1970's. Many, if not most, especially of the poorer Puerto Ricans, lived in 'substandard housing units' (shacks). It was among these people also—perhaps because they had the least—that socialism/communism had the most appeal. Red and black (socialist/independence) flags were prominently displayed in these areas commonly referred to as "barrios."

THE TOWER OF BABEL

One of our early jobs involved cleaning the slats on the inside of a large cooling tower which was about 120 feet high. When we got there the job had already been set up: ropes, electrical cords, and hoses had been strung from the pump truck up to the top entrance area; gauges and control devices were in place. We were carefully watched by Puerto Rican 'eyes' as we 'just off the plane' climbed up to the tower top and into the open slat areas. (I had a fear of heights but I did not show it. We all made it, my fear subsided, and the Puerto Ricans were convinced we were each just like the rest of the gringos. Henceforth, we would be accepted.

The job continued for most of two weeks at night. Commands shouted in English were answered in Spanish. Finally we tried exchanging some Latin and sign language. Inside the mostly darkened cooling tower everything echoed, giving a special effect to the confusion.

But, the job got done. And many more adventures in wet, dirt, grime, height, electric shocks, and exploding gauges/metal hoses followed in the next weeks.

Initially many of the Puerto Ricans (more so than the gringos) were not machinery-oriented. So, there tended to be many more (and more serious) injuries among them than among us. But, more and more, the "Ricans" caught on, man by man.

WE MEET TWO TRINIDADIANS

Just after the beginning we North Americans worked nights (12 hour shifts) and the Puerto Rican crew worked days. One morning after a hard night's work, we stopped at a restaurant/bar often frequented by other North Americans on the Island for *cafe con leche*, a Latin coffee made with strong beans and evaporated milk. It was an inexpensive pick-me-up to keep us awake long enough afterwards to do our laundry—which because of the dirtiness of the work had to be done every morning before going to bed.

At the restaurant that morning two young black men approached us in conversation. Clearly, they wanted to make friends . . .

They told us they were brothers from a middle-class family in Trinidad. They had come to Puerto Rico seeking and finding work as welders. They lived in a shanty on the beach—all they could currently afford—and hoped to better themselves in the long run by coming here . . .

They appeared somehow scared though.

We deduced they were lonely in Puerto Rico and leery of the "Ricans" (many of whom—like many Latins of the era—*hated* blacks). There was no denying these two were nearly 'as black as the ace of spades'.

We considered their unabashed approach. They seemed OK as people and after a bit more conversation the foreman (and us) extended to them our friendship (and thereby our protection)

Soon afterwards we departed for our place.

RAFAEL COLLECTS HIS DEBT

Rafael and Carlos were friends. One day Carlos came to work badly beaten with a black eye. We inquired what had happened. Carlos said he had borrowed $20 from Rafael but Carlos could not pay it back. So, he let Rafael "take it out on him in trade" (beat him up).

"Oh." we said (What could we say?). Both were still friends however, and both would work that day.

TRACY AND I JOURNEY TO UDUADO

The guys had been talking that 'gringos' were rumored to be unwelcome in the Interior of the Island without 'communist' escort. Tracy and I were curious. Our first day off, we took the truck up to Uduado. This town, where we were told the group that tried to assassinate President Truman had originated, had the worst reputation. On the way up we picked up an older Puerto Rican hitchhiker (Tracy told me later it was insurance—unfriendly people would not mess with us if we had local escort) and later dropped him off at his destination. The man was friendly to us however, and at a stop at a fruit stand along the way, showed us the glory of fresh citrus—it is sweet, not bitter. Even the lemons tasted sweet.

Getting to Uduado, we visited the central plaza of the *municipio* with no incident. Then we returned the same day to Ponce. We did discuss beforehand and agree to return to our place by nightfall . . . Occasionally, we had heard that on the narrow winding roads at night, communist cells would threaten to throw up barricades. (I don't know of this actually happening—but it was a verbal harassment technique used against gringos, terrifying motorists, particularly North American tourists and touring U. S. soldiers—thereby discouraging such visits to the Interior and encouraging the belief among whoever they could that it was necessary to discuss matters with them who favored Puerto Rican independence, as well as with the local government officials, most of whom favored statehood or continued Commonwealth status.

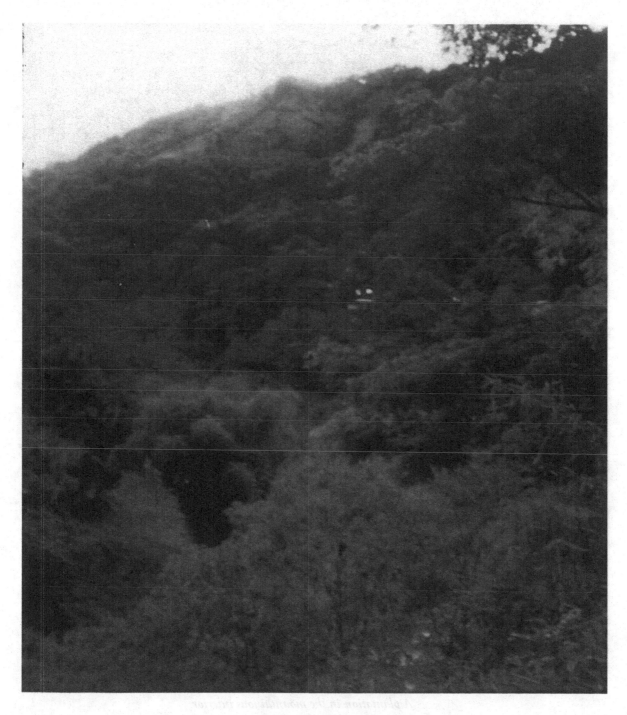

Tropical rain forest near San Juan

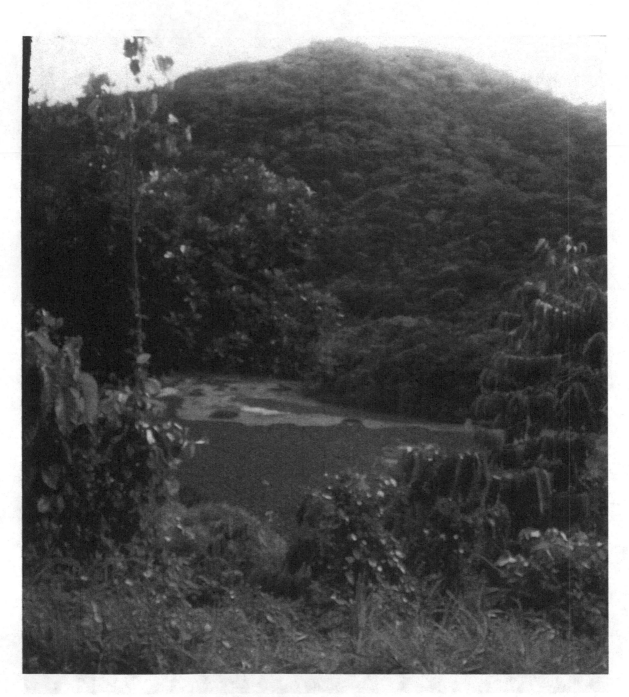

A plantation in the mountainous interior

WE VISIT THE TRINIDADIANS' HUT ON THE BEACH

Meanwhile, one of the Trinidadian brothers, finally trusting our foreman to believe what he was saying, spoke up on the not really inconsiderable matter that was really bothering both of them:

"There is a Soviet soldier living in our house."

"We have no locks on the doors. About two weeks ago, he came up from the beach and came in on us into our house in the night. He came in, his big gun pointed at us."

"We told him (in Spanish) that we were Trinidadians. He said: 'Bueno'."

"He then told us he had deserted his unit in Cuba and made it by boat to Puerto Rico."

"He eats our food (and we don't have much to share). He wears our clothes. He sleeps at our place. He never leaves. He snaps at us. He has stashed his loaded gun in our closet."

"He says he wants to talk to some Americans. He says he wants to 'come over,' but he doesn't want to get shot."

"Can you guys meet with him and help him turn himself in? This would make us very happy."

The foreman broke the news to us when he next saw us at our place. It was late in the afternoon. Having worked all night the night before, we had just gotten up.

It was at that point that four wide-eyed young Americans with differing perspectives and personal backgrounds simultaneously thought the same thought:

"What is an armed Soviet soldier doing on U.S. soil?" The need to investigate was clear.

Rick, our resident Vietnam vet, softly popped a direct question: "Where is his gun?" (Rick always spoke softly since a piercing bullet had damaged part of his vocal chords in Vietnam.)

The foreman said that he told the Trinidadians that before we meet with this Soviet, he must beach his gun at least 500 yards from the hut. He is awaiting their assurance that this condition has been met. Then, we can meet with him.

This sounded logical and was OK with all. We agreed to all go together and prepared to do so.

Soon afterward the foreman went out in the truck. He came back as it was getting dark. He said: "Let's go."

He drove the van. Rick sat in the front seat with him. We other three piled into the back of the van. All together we headed over the street system for the Trinidadians' shanty on the beach.

Thusly, we left on our mission of peace . . .

HISTORICAL NOTE: It was my understanding that an armed Soviet soldier in uniform on U.S. soil was a fair target for our military. A Russian soldier out of uniform could be regarded by our military as a spy. Soviet deserters if returned to their communist government were summarily shot. He was in a three-way *dilemma*

FACE-TO-FACE WITH AN UNCAPTURED SOVIET SOLDIER/ DESERTER: WE WERE UNARMED . . .

Soon we were there. As we emptied out of the van I briefly thought to myself, shouldn't we fan out just in case he didn't do as agreed? But, I perished the thought. It would sound weak and probably look even worse if I were to say that. I quietly gritted my teeth and with the others boldly walked in the wide open to the entrance of the shack.

One of the Trinidadians appeared at the door and motioned us to come in.

We entered the 'front room' where none of us had ever been before. It had a dirt floor, one light bulb was suspended from the ceiling. The bulb provided the only light. There was no furniture except some wooden crates to sit on. Now, we were inside, hidden from the outside . . .

Suddenly, the foreman burst out in an anguished tone: "Where is he?" (If betrayed at this point, we were now perfectly set up to be slaughtered, and perhaps buried in the 'tomb of the unknown civilians'.)

Immediately, however, the other black brother appeared at the interior door across the front room, followed by the Soviet. They walked in and nodded.

We nodded back and all then sat down too, squatted or seated in a rough semi-circle on the dirt floor under the light of the single light bulb.

The Soviet was average sized, age about 23 to 28, somewhat scuzzy-looking, and dressed in civilian clothes that didn't fit him right. But, best of all, he was unarmed—we immediately noted!

The Trinidadian who had led the Soviet into the room with us told us that the soldier spoke only some Russian languages and limited Spanish. He, the Trinidadian, since he spoke Spanish and English, would act as interpreter.

For once in my life I had the presence of mind to keep my mouth entirely shut. I sat eagle-eyed with the three other eagle-eyed gringos a few feet from the Soviet and the others: the black Trinidadians and our foreman.

As a gesture of peace someone lit up a square and passed it around. Everyone took a drag including the Soviet.

> **HISTORICAL NOTE:** In those days passing around a lit cigarette was a recognized gesture of peace in both the Soviet Union and the United States. Technically healthy or not, it seemed appropriate in this circumstance...

Point made. We could begin our meeting.

The foreman questioned the Soviet. His questions were translated into Spanish by the interpreting black Trinidadian. The Soviet's answers were spoken to the Trinidadian in Spanish and translated by the black to us in English.

The Soviet's answers were short and clipped.

Our eyes studied his reactions and his eyes with intent . . . If he'd made a fearful or hostile movement toward the ulterior door, all four of us quiet ones would have tackled him . . . How trustworthy is a desperate deserter? (Whether "freedom-seeking" or not?)

However, we learned:

He sincerely wanted to come over.

He had deserted his unit stationed in Cuba.

He was a combat soldier (trained in combat and part of a combat unit).

He had made it to Puerto Rico (apparently by boat or raft) all the way from Cuba.

He wanted peace.

He learned:

He must turn himself in soon.

We would make some arrangements to expedite.

We would give him some time to get himself together. (We would not citizens' arrest him tonight.)

We wanted peace, too.

Enough said, the meeting broke up and we departed back to our place in the van.

Later the foreman indicated the Soviet had been turned in at the police department (because of the gun) and was "welcomed" by immigration authorities and the U. S. Army. By the way, the foreman continued that the Trinidadians in their haste to arrange a turnover and not alienate their uninvited 'guest' had lied to us about the whereabouts of the gun: it was in the kitchen closet when we were all there.

No public mention of this was made at the time and we were told to simply forget about it because of the Cold War. When the government did finally in a politically timed announcement put notice in the U.S. papers admitting the presence of a Soviet combat unit in Cuba (1977), I speculated if this Soviet had been a help to them on the matter.

NOTE: The government knows many things long before they tell the public.

THE DECISION TO LEAVE PUERTO RICO

Finally, one day soon afterwards, covered in wet carbon black from head to foot working at an area plant, and getting a bit tired of living in close quarters, (There were now 6 of us in the place.), I decided to explore working for one of the plants down there and get my own place. I talked to a local personnel manager and he welcomed the idea of an educated gringo worker. But, I had no skills except hydrocleaning and office skills (These were not needed and I was not fluent in Spanish.) Soon, I decided to return stateside and get a job in my field of geography.

THE RETURN STATESIDE AND REFLECTIONS ON THE CARIBBEAN SEA

Flying high over the Caribbean Sea during the return stateside, I left Puerto Rico feeling much better about myself than I had in recent months. The exercise and challenge, though short-lived, had significantly repaired my shattered self-image (due to being psychologically unfit for military service despite my father's attempts to toughen me up).

When at Christmas 1990, the Cold War ended and I was 'down on myself for not really having done much, suddenly this memory of the Soviet flashed up in my weird mind . . . It all came back THEN. Though I hadn't done much, I had done something.

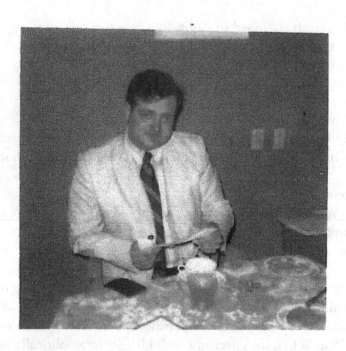

A young Ron Doyle returned home safely,
glad he made the work trip but happy to be home

POSTSCRIPT

Even after returning from Puerto Rico I continued to have difficulty performing well on jobs. The last job in the series of jobs during these unhappy times was as an airport limousine driver. I drove for the cab company while an employment agency, looked for a job as a geographer for me.

There was only one incident . . . It occurred one day when a child kidnapper rented my cab at the airport. He had me take him in my cab to nearby Belpre where he left the cab to try to kidnap his child from his ex-wife's house. While he was 'doing his thing' I contacted my dispatcher on the cab radio and the police quickly came and took him into custody. I made out a police report.

After three months on this job a telephone call prompted me to an interview in Cleveland . . .

(In Cleveland I finally connected with a job I could do fairly well for an extended period of time despite my disabilities, and for the following fourteen years worked all over North America as a professional geographer and facility location consultant. But, that's another story for another chapter . . .)

APPENDIX

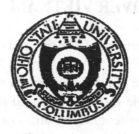

THE RETURN TO OSU

CAPTURING MY BACHELOR'S DEGREE

Coming off the job with Lazarus (Federated Dept. Stores) where I worked as an order picker in their warehouse during the Christmas season of 1968, I re-undertook studies at OSU beginning Winter Quarter '69 with a minimal fulltime load. Brent Demlow, my male nurse friend from Harding, continued to encourage me and talk me through resuming the routine at school all through both winter and spring of '69. The 'new Ronnie' was still a good student but decidedly slower and more limited than before the mental attacks of last spring, in due course, I graduated in June of '69 with my Bachelor of Arts Degree in Geography with no special distinction.

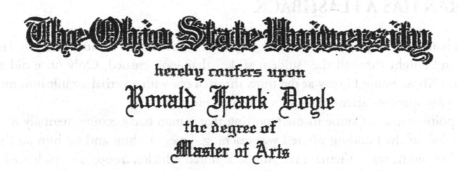

OSU GRAD SCHOOL

BEGINNING STUDIES FOR MY MASTER'S DEGREE

I finished up my summer work with C.H. Heist Corporation and returned to Columbus toward Fall '69 to begin studies for a Master's Degree in Geography, the recipient of a teaching assistantship. While I studied I also taught undergraduate geography laboratories for the next two years at the Columbus campus.

THE NATIONAL DEBATE OVER VIETNAM COMES TO CAMPUS

By spring 1970 the national concern over Vietnam (and other issues) had burst onto campuses of the land.

The pattern was simple: legitimate peace supporters, as well as self-interested radical elements would come onto the campuses, mingle with the interested students, and organize demonstrations sympathetic to ending the U. S. involvement in Vietnam. The peace groups strove to leave it at that, gaining impact (with the public and the Congress) from TV exposure. The radicals, however, sought to then turn the demonstrations toward violence and disarray, assisting their agenda of national disruption. I sympathized with the positive virtues of those who wanted to save me, themselves, and others from the war and through my network of family and friends always defended their virtues with words of support for them. Many of the 'peace people' themselves were Vietnam veterans or veterans of earlier wars. The churches were heavily involved.

However, some of the radicals were not on the "peace" side of Congress, or even on the side of the 'land and people of the United States'. As I convivially penetrated the peace-seeking circles at OSU, I learned of two Cuban soldiers "touring" the area from a woman I had just met in the crowd. But, when I questioned her about them, she quickly evaded me and slipped away. I never did find out where these two were being hidden. I was not of a mind to be protective of these intervening "non-interventionists" for I wondered if these were the same Cuban soldiers who had threatened a bomb blast at my MOBAY workplace during the last summer.

[Meanwhile, as I was milling around the students and others, 15,000 National Guardsmen arrived in armored columns, and thousands of police, to keep order.]

A VETERAN HAS A FLASHBACK

As a graduate teaching assistant—and an employee of the State of Ohio—I honored my contract with OSU and taught through the "student strike" that soon ensued. Only once did a 'striker,' a black militant whose name I knew at the time, threaten me with a verbal assault into my classroom window. But my students attending classes defended me.

At one point a student came to me reporting that a man had become mentally disoriented in the entrance hall of the building where I was teaching. I went to him and sat him on the steps and listened . . . He said he was a Vietnam vet. All the armored vehicles, troops, and violence had brought memories back! I looked directly into his eyes, got his attention, and spoke to him softly saying that he was not the target here! These are demonstrating students, they have no guns! The National Guardsmen have all the guns. This seemed to register with him and he became calm again.

GASSED!

At some risk to myself and with only the authorization that comes with being alive in a troubled zone, as the demonstrations headed toward more physical confrontation, I went into the peopled areas and started taking pictures left and right as one of many instructors who in those days tried to head off campus violence by intimidating potential wrongdoers with the power of a camera.

> **HISTORICAL NOTE:** There was a saying at the time: "The left is the right." They work in tandem to create instability. Not everyone who said they favored the Vietnam War escalation policy actually was in favor of it. Not everyone opposed was truthfully opposed. Enough said. Know the people. Talk is misleading—study actions, motives . . .

SPRING BREAK 1970

Ultimately the efforts of the peacekeepers, including the picture takers (like myself) and others who wanted peace on campus, failed, as 'the radical left and the militant right' succeeded in their ambitions to create conditions unsafe enough to warrant closing the university. I was on the side of the spirit of the law . . . This permitted dissent (from the law) or affirmation (agreement with the law), but not breaking the laws.

The radicals were dispersed. Some arrests were made. The undergraduates were all sent home as the undergraduate school was closed. (It had been an undergraduate strike/demonstration that had been called). I stayed on with the rest of the graduate students and finished up the quarter. I then left the campus for the summer.

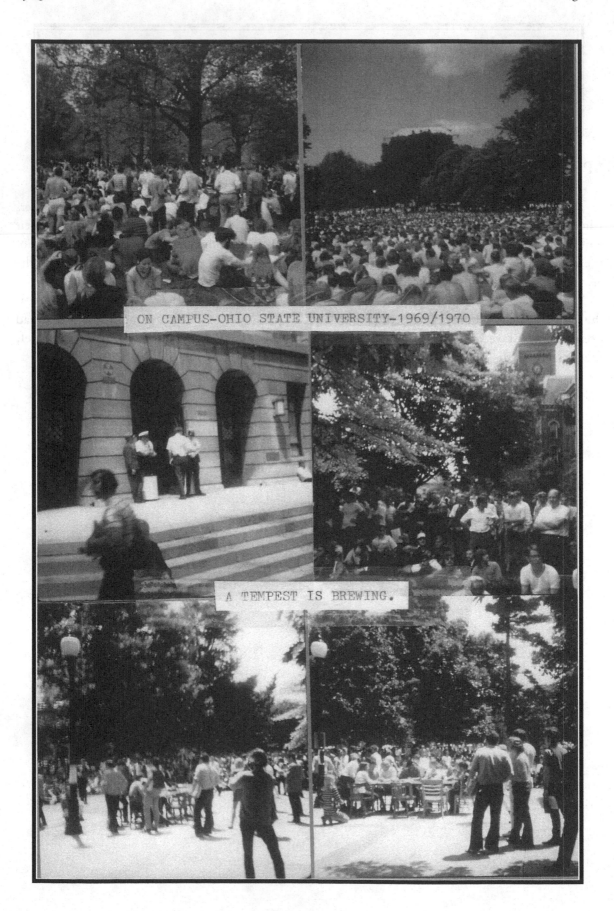

ON CAMPUS—OHIO STATE UNIVERSITY—1969/1970

A TEMPEST IS BREWING.

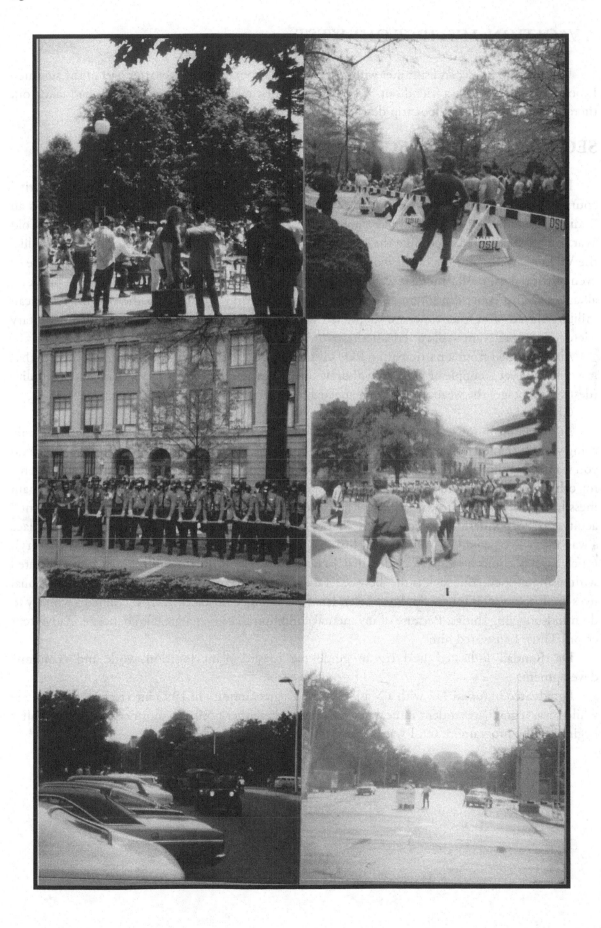

A VACATION: MY FIRST OUT WEST

Finishing up my second summer with C. H. Heist Corporation, in the latter part of the summer, I took a trip by car with a friend out West. It was the first major trip this geographer had taken out there. The highlight was a foot trip down to the base of the Grand Canyon.

SECOND YEAR GRAD SCHOOL: 1970-1971

I returned to OSU and to studying/part-time teaching in the fall. I took a 'national security' course under Dr. Randall, a former OSS officer and geographer, called 'political geography,' as an 'individual studies' option. I learned among other things that although publicly during the Cold War, America postured itself 'like the Romans' (Pax Americana), our basic strategy was really 'like the Vikings'. With only 7% of the world's population, we did not in this country seek world rule or even territorial gain. All America's wars and other military actions were designed as raids, to break up alliances against American interests. Sometimes, as after World War II, after the raid the American military stayed on. Other times we simply left when the necessity of being 'there' ended. (Military 'victory' is not relevant—all American actions are 'search and destroy' raids.)

Also I learned from a participating ROTC student soon to graduate and become an officer that it would take yet 'a couple of years' to withdraw the U.S. Armed Forces from Vietnam and neutralize (destroy/sabotage) the weapons systems expected to be left behind.

Glum news . . .

At one point in my training Dr. Randall pointedly cornered me, saying: "Doyle, about the only thing you are trained for as a geographer is war policy planning or plant location planning. Which do you want?" I at this time did not like the concept of war, did not like the idea of planning such events for others either—and did not envision the opportunity to do war planning better. (The Vietnam mess had turned me off to that career.) I had also thought at the time to not trust my own mental acuity too. So, pondering the worst case scenario, I reasoned that if I helped to inadvertently misplace a war, many lives would be unnecessarily lost. If I helped to inadvertently mislocate a plant (factory), much money could be lost. I decided that I could better live with the guilt and shame associated with losing money. (But such is the 'between a rock and a hard place' syndrome of most professional lives . . . Either way is tough. And, sooner or later, there will be mistakes made by humans who try to do mind-boggling things. Because of my mental condition there was a greater chance of inadvertent error.) Thus, I answered him.

Dr. Randall indicated he'd try to guide me toward plant location work and economic development.

I graduated in June 1971 with a Master of Arts Degree. Inquiry in 1993 into records made of me while I was a graduate student indicated I was unnoted: neither positively nor negatively noted after beginning the program in '69. I was lackluster—but not irresponsible.

B-176

DOYLE, RONALD FRANK, B.A.	THE OHIO STATE UNIVERS
Name	COLUMBUS, OHIO
	OFFICE OF THE REGISTRAR

Permanent Student Number

VIENNA, WEST VIRGINIA   MAY 2, 1946
Address   Date of Birth

VINCENT LEO DOYLE   VIENNA, WEST VIRGINIA
Parent, Guardian, or Spouse   Address

Admission Information	Title of Course	Department	Course Number	Cr. Hrs.	Grade	Pts.
	TRANSFERRED FROM ARTS TO GRADUATE SCHOOL OCTOBER 1969					
	AUTUMN QUARTER 1969					
B.A.	APPL QUANT METH 1	GEOG	883.01	4	B	12
THE OHIO	SEMINARS	GEOG	889	5	B	15
STATE	COMPOSITION 1	GERMAN	204	2*	E	0
UNIVERSITY						
JUNE 1969	**WINTER QUARTER 1970**					
	INT MICRO-EC THRY	ECON	501	4	A	16
	APPL QUANT METH 2	GEOG	883.02	4	B	12
	SEMINARS	GEOG	889	5	B	15
	SPRING QUARTER 1970					
	SPECIAL STUDIES	ECON	694	4	A16	
	GROUP STUDIES	GEOG	694	5	B15	
	THRY OF URBAN GEOG	GEOG	850.01	5	S	
	AUTUMN QUARTER 1970					
	INDIVIDUAL STUDIES	GEOG	693	3	S	
	INDIVIDUAL STUDIES	GEOG	693	5	S	
	WINTER QUARTER 1971					
	GEOG OF DEVELOPMNT	GEOG	642	5	B	15
	PROBS IN URBN GEOG	GEOG	850.02	5	A20	
	SPRING QUARTER 1971					
	GROUP STUDIES	GEOG	694	5	B	15
	THRY OF URBAN GEOG	GEOG	850.01	5	B	15

*NOT FOR GRADUATE CREDIT

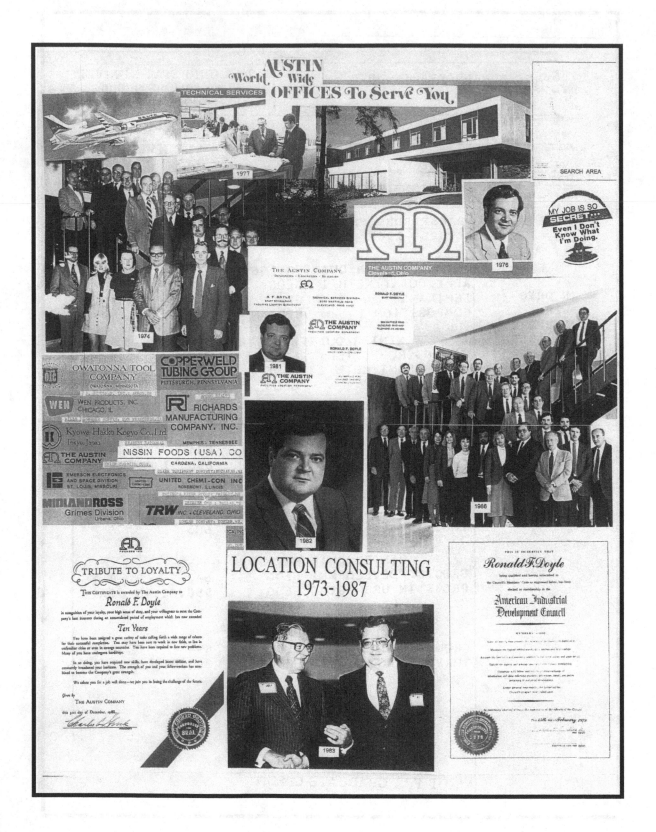

CHAPTER FOUR

SOARING WITH EAGLES

In Recovery: My Brief Career as a Professional Geographer
(1973-1987): 22% OF MY LIFE BEFORE AGE 62

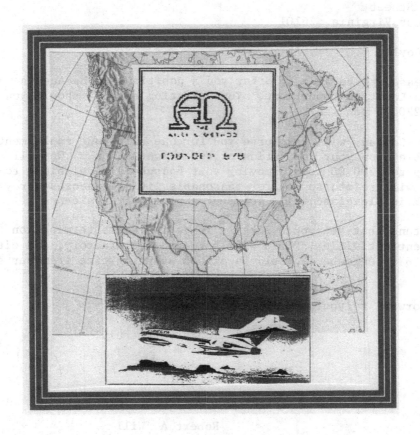

A BRIEF CAREER:

THE AUSTIN COMPANY YEARS

OFFICES IN PRINCIPAL CITIES

THE AUSTIN COMPANY

DESIGNERS · ENGINEERS · BUILDERS

3650 MAYFIELD ROAD · CLEVELAND, OHIO 44121

FOUNDED 1878

November 7, 1973

Mr. Ronald E. Doyle
1004 44th Street
Vienna, West Virginia 26101

Dear Mr. Doyle:

We are pleased to be able to offer you a position in The Austin Company's Facilities Location Department. Your starting salary, should you accept, will be $220.00 per week.

The Austin Company will reimburse you for one-half your employment agency fee, payable upon your completion of three months work. We will also provide up to $200.00 toward moving your household furnishings to Cleveland, and will reimburse you for reasonable living expenses for your first week in Cleveland while you seek a permanent residence.

We understand that you would like at least two weeks termination time for your present activities. This will be quite satisfactory, and either November 26 or December 3 would be a good starting time from our standpoint.

We look forward to your reply.

Yours very truly,

Robert A. Will
Manager
Facilities Location Department

RAW: gm

JOB DESCRIPTION

STAFF CONSULTANT - FACILITIES LOCATION DEPARTMENT

REPORTS TO: Department Manager

BASIC FUNCTION: To comparatively evaluate potential locations for a client's proposed operation and to recommend those locations judged as most satisfactorily meeting the operation's requirements.

MAJOR RESPONSIBILITIES AND KEY DUTIES:

a. Assume responsibility for performing the study analysis, reviewing analysis and developing conclusions/recommendations with department manager, supervising graphic and secretarial support staff in production of report, and presenting recommendations to client.

b. Review operating requirements for proposed operation and research data from in-house files or from outside sources to evaluate tangible cost factors (i.e., transportation, labor, taxes, utilities, etc.) and intangible considerations (i.e., quality of life, labor climate, etc.) in order to determine the most favorable sector of the study area for the proposed operation.

c. Field visit the selected candidate locations within the recommended favorable area to obtain current information on conditions related to the operating requirements of the proposed operation to determine the most favorable locations.

d. Prepare the tables, exhibits and narrative report needed to present the analysis and support the conclusions/recommendations of the study.

e. Participate in presentation meeting with client to review analysis, conclusions and recommendations.

f. Coordinate the work assignments to the support staff with other department consultants to facilitate preparation of report tables, exhibits and narrative text.

g. Coordinate analysis needs/problems, study progress, analysis results/conclusions, field condition observations, and client comments/inquiries with the department manager.

h. Coordinate study progress and client presentation meetings with the company's sales representative to assure his informed status and permit his attendance at client meetings.

i. Accompany client representatives on tour of recommended location.

j. Obtain option on selected property and arrange for soil/ foundation exploration, title search, zoning changes and other needed services to facilitate client's final evaluation and program implementation.

k. Fulfill these responsibilities and key duties in recognition of the authorized scope, budget, schedule and the department's quality standards.

l. Coordinate analysis data, conclusions, problems and opportunities, especially field observations, with other department consultants to assure exchange of current information.

m. Stay abreast of professional field and assist in developing and maintaining current data base for study analysis, especially for newly emerging or changing basic considerations.

n. Encourage and assist in development of other department consultants and support staff.

o. Represent The Austin Company at client meetings and field visits in a professional and complimentary manner.

* * * * * *

A REQUIREMENT OF EACH STUDY:

"The study will be conducted confidentially without revealing the name of the Client."

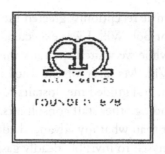

A BRIEF CAREER

AS A GEOGRAPHER

In December 1973 I became a staff consultant at The Austin Company (Cleveland) doing facility location studies for Fortune 500 companies who were Austin s clients. My life became a little more stable . . .

I spent the next 14 years (1973-1987) at The Austin Company, headquartered in Cleveland. I travelled the airways, highways, and byways of North America (U.S., Canada, Mexico) looking for sites suitable to recommend for specific client industrial and miscellaneous facilities. I worked as the project engineer (team man in the field) on over 50 location projects. I easily visited 1000 communities interviewing their representatives, plant representatives, other leaders, and taking notes, making analyses and reports. Output to be produced by the plants ranged the gamut from defense products, capital goods equipment, consumer durables, foods, and information. Overall, working for the Austin Company was a positive experience for me.

I lived in apartments of progressively better quality as my income from my employment rose. My last apartment was directly on the lake, overlooking Lake Erie from 17 floors up. It had a panoramic view of the lake and sunsets over the water were exquisitely beautiful. But, I was hardly ever at my place to enjoy it: these were years of travel, job stress, and rush on company business, barhopping for social entertainment (people-watching), conversation, and alcoholic sedative, and retrospectively unwise involvement with other people and their mental problems or problems with the law. Stresses mounted and my mental health problems sporadically resurfaced. Cleveland relationships overall I therefore remember as a less positive experience than working for The Austin Company.

Ultimately, I burned out like a light bulb! Then one day, it was just time to leave as I perceived clouds gathering over me as social relationships mysteriously deteriorated, and, suddenly, my employment terminated. After a simultaneously occurring hospital operation (gall bladder), I headed back to the hills'. My brother drove the truck with all my belongings in it. My parents drove their car with me riding (not yet recovered from surgery) in the back seat.

THE PROFESSIONAL GEOGRAPHER

I walked past the beautiful gardens of the area in front of the headquarters building of The Austin Company, a moderate-sized impressive award-winning architectural structure of marble and glass. A well dressed, well-spoken female receptionist greeted me at the desk and upon my giving her my name, she telephoned upstairs for Bob Will. I was expected.

The lobby was impressive and while we waited she took me on a guided tour of the "corporate history" room. Soon, Robert A. Will, Manager of the Facilities Location Department, arrived, engaged me in pleasant conversation, and guided me upstairs to the General Department.

I talked with several people including other staff consultants. I had few questions as I needed the job. This job already appeared better than what my advanced education had gotten me so far: better than cleaning sewers and exposing myself to invisible deadly gasses, better even teaching in a ghetto school, more favorable than working in a (at the time) sporadically unpredictable Spanish-speaking area far from home, or even working, covered by assassination insurance, for local political bureaucrats who despised me.

The Austin people had several questions of me. Apparently, I answered them satisfactorily . . . That interview went awfully easily though. No matter, I needed work . . .

Upon acceptance of The Austin Company's offer, I rented an upstairs apartment on Buxton Road in South Euclid, moved in as much foldable furniture as I could pack into my car, and began work at The Austin Company December 3, 1973.

The General Department consisted of a small group of young plant location consultants (a mix of professional geographers and engineers), and a larger group of generally older senior consultants, each of whom was a renowned expert in a field or several fields related to the construction industry. The senior consultants were "above" me in knowledge and experience without question. I was somewhat awed by them. Of course, I never showed them that!

(In Cleveland, throughout the corporate culture, smart men cooped up at times in the office play nasty games with young professionals. It's not malice usually, just amusement for highly stimulated talented minds that despite even huge project loads need more to keep them fully occupied. I did not wish to open myself up to be the turkey at a turkey shoot so I played their sparring games with them as carefully as I could. But, a verbal knife in the back with a full twist—this started about the end of the first week—has to be returned convincingly, but with friendliness. Otherwise, they make a case against you. (This process continued throughout my professional life there.)

The corporate religion was "conservativism," the corporate party appeared to be GOP. When I first came there the office was decorated in shades of gray and black with a large clock on the central front wall. Desks were arranged in rows in a bull pen. Managers watched from inside glass enclosures. The pace was strong, steady. Day began at 8:30 AM sharp punctually. Lunch commenced in groups at 12 and everyone returned to the office (and began work) at 1 PM. They laid down their pencils at 5:30 PM. By 5:40 PM, the corporate parking lot was vacated except for the cars of those worked overtime. Nixon was still President. The thinking was "somewhat to the right of Attila the Hun, who himself, was rumored to have been a too tolerant sissy".

I had long hair (Buster Brown style), spoke 'Democratese,' and delighted in doing my charts in colored pens. I was brazenly thought-provoking . . . (I was however noticed).

They watched my work carefully . . . I was slowly accepted (I hoped actions spoke louder than words/symbols with this highly educated group). But there was a lot of gamey sparring with the old men. We needed to come together I needed accepted, they needed for me to *change and grow* at least some, for I had been weakened more than I at that time had realized by the 1968-1973 traumatic period in my life.

Also, I was still on the pills: dependent on anti-psychotic medications that fought off severe mind alteration episodes, but which themselves caused some reality perception gaps.

The job itself was perfect: my work was thoroughly checked, mistakes caught work often judged and positively criticized. Wisdom and strength began to take positive form in my work. But, a not inconsiderable problem arose, that plagued me throughout my career. Because of my condition, and the importance that my details as well as conclusions be right, often I would be over-revealing about my doubtful judgments on projects leaving the impression that I 'lacked self-confidence'. It wasn't self-confidence that I lacked. It was a fully functioning brain that I missed. (I leaned on everybody heavily as reality checks. This is dangerous in the corporate culture because office politics will always be played).

But given the only two options I had (to reveal possible mistakes or to keep my mouth shut) I did the professional thing. While I was there, my work would be as right as I could (with others) make it.

Socially, I kept a very low profile. Mostly, I stayed to myself.

But, I did frequent area bars engaging in conversations with mostly strangers, sampling what truths I could from them get as reality checks. Often, strangers opened up quicker than people I knew (for they knew or believed we would not see each other again).

Unfortunately, there was an often significant negative side to this approach—I learned to talk fast and have ready proof that I was kidding or lying about some things I said to them in order to get them to open up to me.

Psychiatrically, it was a period of great variability. At night I often had "eyes-open" illusions of my body floating off the bed toward the ceiling, and many other weird (disease and prescription drug caused) sensations. These things were not actually happening (I checked), just my brain chemistry kept a continual stream of strange things being perceived. Sleeping was usually difficult . . . mornings continued to come too soon.

But, time would soon reveal that the job was what my young geographer's heart had always pined for. It was a geographer's position within "the military-industrial complex" which served the U. S. military, many FORTUNE 500 companies, and several multi-nationals.

I had a staff position with the location department as a location consultant for new facility locations of our clients. It was a small job, but interesting.

ROBERT A. WILL

My first 'leader' was the department manager, Robert A. Will. Excellent with people, he had a 'dutch uncle' management style. It was a pleasure to work for him and I learned much from him as my stamina built up to work on many projects.

And many projects ensued . . . (See PROJECT NOTES AND HIGHLIGHTS (1973-1976))

By February 1976 I was ready for a vacation. I returned to the Ponce area for a week in the sun. Staying at the Holiday Inn, the highlight was a dinner with another tourist (a real estate woman) and her husband Puerto Rican style with a local businessman at his house, and a trip by myself by car back up into the interior to see if there had been any changes . . .

In August, I was hospitalized for a "schizophrenic reaction" as feeling my confidence surge I withdrew too soon from the medication . . . I returned to work in a month or so and was able at this time to recover quite quickly.

1976 was the year of the post-Vietnam presidential election. I strongly identified with the Democrats then and many diverse conversations ensued at the office. In this highly Republican atmosphere I would have been better served by simply keeping my mouth shut.

Differing concepts of national affairs solutions aside, I associated often socially with many of the "conservatives" at the office, and at social affairs of the Company—especially with Kondik.

His little group called themselves "the bad boys". I thought they were "good boys," even though most differed with my viewpoints. To them, I admittedly must have been hard for them to figure: I'm sure they thought I was a satan . . . They dubbed me "the General" (a diminutive) and stuck me with that name (for I did talk excessively on and on). I got a kick out of pretending to be a radical. In this highly conservative company it raised eyebrows. In fact, though I carried on only in conversation with them and in immediate social circles. I had no political organizational contacts—I talked as often as not with sardonic humor . . . I was pro-American (my actions on the job at my work and sacrifices I readily made for the corporate and the national interests showed that). Policy matters aside, I was for the American spirit of the law (as I understood it).

Nevertheless, I was a 'suspicious' person to them.

But, it was Kondik who got arrested toward the last days of the Ford regime. In 1976, he and several of his neighbors were arrested and prosecuted for petition fraud. Trials followed.

STEVE APPLEBY

Steve Appleby became manager in 1976. His management style tended to keep all of his people 'off-balance'. He seemed to me to vary in moods from "The Sun King' (who could make one feel top of the world), then later, he would be 'The Dark Side of the Moon'. Then, revert back . . . This technique pushes and strains, gets out the production, but my body and mind eventually revolted against me (and sometimes him also!) However, I was determined to survive in my job and did so for the challenge . . . I succeeded, but at a serious cost of strains not properly handled (because I did not know how to handle stress well.)

On the positive side though, he was able to get enough work flowing into the department to keep several staff consultants, including me, very busy. Many interesting projects ensued . . . (See PROJECT NOTES AND HIGHLIGHTS (1976-1984)). I worked fairly hard and steady with much travelling and often tight schedules . . .

After the Reagan landslide of 1980, gradually the Republicans consolidated their hold on everything important to my life at the time . . . Democrats (who were not even welcome on the Joint Chiefs of Staff nor in most high military or *civilian* positions) became low profile at the company, too. My loyalty transferred to the new Supreme War Authority, Ronald Reagan, the President, as a matter of citizenship. I began aping some of his type of thinking . . . but still doubted that political party.

By 1982, however, my salary now reasonably high, and having been recently made a stockholder (part owner and now a "principal employee") of the old privately held Austin Company, I moved into a luxury apartment in the Watergate complex in Euclid. Seventeen floors up (lakeside at the point) my apartment had a commanding view of the lake looking out every window. Sunsets on the watery horizon were particularly gorgeous.

Of course, when companies pay you enough to have all these accoutrements, they think they own you (And they do . . .). I was never there. I was on the road for the company. The apartment mostly was empty—it was a storage space for my carefully arranged furniture and increasing amounts of gear.

But sometimes when I was in town, it was beautiful living.

Also, now at a more sensitive level (money-wise) there was more visibility and exposure to the upper management, adding up in these recessionary times to less job security. But I was getting older and older—I had never had job security. What is that anyway?

One only lives once. I enjoyed the gusto . . .

Also during this year I went to Mexico on brief vacation.

Meanwhile at work, things slowed down to a crawl and I was shortly laid off. The layoff was temporary though and within six weeks I was b.tck on full time.

The office talk centered around "guns" in the emerging face off with the U.S.S.R.: the side with the most and best guns properly deployed dynamically wins! America was no longer conducting a multi-faceted global effort (economic, political, informational, etc.) against the Soviets-everything was strictly "guns". The Austin Company's ATS Division was heavily involved in making sophisticated weapons systems for the military, (as all along we had been), and I was involved on some defense plant location work (Nothing new for me).

Seeing some of these weapons systems as they were developed at work familiarized me with the military arms potentials of the era. (But I never had, nor did I ever want personal access to these systems.)

Meanwhile, project work resumed with brief interruptions. I had steady employment and mostly steady work until the end of Steve's reign.

JAMES BOONE

In 1984, Jim Boone and I were evaluated for the location department's manager position as Steve departed for an assignment in National Gypsum, our new owner. I did not actively seek the position, but was surprised when I didn't get it. In retrospect, the company had decided correctly though as I was dim-minded again more than I realized . . . due to the long period of heavy project work as well as my *by now regrettable* involvement with Kondik. Pleasantly though, my title was upgraded to recognize my long service and my salary stayed quite high. Jim's management technique at the time was young and benign.

Due this time to the strain being suddenly removed (and other reasons), I collapsed in February and was hospitalized for 10 days in the psychiatric ward of a local hospital.

It was months before I was working at minimally acceptable levels again in my job. And after this episode, I gradually waned in clearheaded mental strength . . .

This became increasingly noticeable by others . . . As my brief career wound down toward an end many projects still ensued (See PROJECT NOTES AND HIGHLIGHTS (1984-1987)).

Finally, I could see that this era in my life was ending . . . I could see the end in Cleveland and began to prepare for it. In July I was told I'd be laid off (permanently). At the same time I developed gall bladder problems . . .

I was laid off from the Austin Company on August 15, 1987 in a "friendly termination". Almost immediately afterward, I entered the hospital for gall bladder surgery.

REFLECTIONS ON THE POND: The Austin Experience

Austin used me up and threw me away . . . But, they gave me many good memories, fourteen years of employment in my chosen field of geography doing things for the national economy and other national good. On balance, I have few complaints (nor am I harboring any), and some fond thoughts about some of the people I once knew there.

"REFLECTIONS ON THE LAKE: The Cleveland Experience

As one coworker said to me about his own experience: "I made lots of money to buy things to impress people who still didn't like me." I found the rat race punishing. Cleveland, on balance at the time was neither welcoming nor offensive, but, as in "Murphy's Law," friends departed and enemies collected. God bless true friendships . . . In all those tries, I made but a few.

DRIVEN BACK INTO THE HILLS

I thus ended my exploration of and crusade in the world (because I had no other choice). I had to end my 'wandering in the desert'. I was not to find the 'Promised Land' in Cleveland.

I simply went back home . . . My 'race' ended, I 'pulled in my oar'.

At the end of August, ray father drove his white Mercury Grand Marquis out of the Watergate parking lot, my mother rode "shotgun" and I, still crippled from the gall bladder operation, sat blanketed in the rear. We headed back into the hills.

Aside from taking care of necessary or legally required business, I never returned to the Cleveland area for many years.

EVALUATIONS

monday

Labor

Speaker: Ronald F. Doyle, Staff Consultant, Facilities Location Department, The Austin Company

10:15 a.m.   **Coffee Break**
Regency Ballroom Foyer

Financing

Speaker: John J. Dues, Director, Corporate Real Estate, The Mead Corporation

Water and Services

Speaker: Steven L. Johnson, Engineer & Hydrologist, Winslow & Associates, Inc.

Question and Answer Session

      Luncheon
Regency Ballroom D

...nes T. Schaefer, President, IDRC,
...e Director of Real Estate, Beatrice
...ny

Hon. David C. Treen, Governor,
...siana

Concurrent Professional Workshop

...VENING

Board Buses for Reception

...ng will start at the Hyatt Motor Lobby
Buses will run on a shuttle basis.

Cocktail Reception
The Cabildo in the French Quarter
...red by the State of Louisiana.

THE INDUSTRIAL DEVELOPMENT RESEARCH COUNCIL, INC.

November 19, 1982

The Austin Company
Ronald F. Doyle
Staff Consultant
1850 Mayfield Drive
Cleveland, Ohio 44121

Dear Ron:

Once again, another rewarding and productive IDRC Professional Seminar has been concluded, and we can look back with pride and satisfaction on a job well done!

The program was outstanding, and we are grateful for your role in creating this success. We thank you for your professional participation in both the planning and the execution of the seminar.

Sincerely,

McKinley Conway
Executive Director

Martin K. Finley
Deputy Director

James D. Mathis
Program Officer

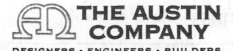

THE AUSTIN COMPANY

DESIGNERS • ENGINEERS • BUILDERS

3650 MAYFIELD ROAD
CLEVELAND, OHIO 44121
TELEPHONE 216/382-6600
TELETYPE 810-421-8540
CABLE: AUSTINCLEGEN

TO WHOM IT MAY CONCERN:

Ronald F. Doyle was employed by The Austin Company from 1973 through August 15, 1987 as a staff consultant in the Facilities Location Department. In 1985, his title was changed from "Location Consultant" to "Senior Location Consultant." In this position, he was responsible for assisting corporate clients in evaluating locations throughout the U. S., Canada and Mexico for proposed manufacturing, distribution, and office operations.

Mr. Doyle has exceptional analytical and research capabilities which were instrumental in the completion of many statistical and computer-related assignments. He recently was a primary participant in formulating an internal company marketing and industry analysis. In addition, he has traveled extensively nationwide and is familiar with varying business conditions in many areas of the United States.

Mr. Doyle has interacted with and assisted management in our client's organization on many occasions and has performed well. He should be a fine addition to any firm needing the above capabilities.

Very truly yours,

Thomas B. Sweeney
Senior Vice President
Design and Engineering

TBS:mg

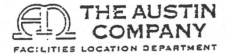

THE AUSTIN COMPANY

FACILITIES LOCATION DEPARTMENT

3650 MAYFIELD ROAD
CLEVELAND, OH 44121
PHONE: 216/382-6600
TELEX 910-421-8540
CABLE AUSTIN

August 14, 1987

Dear Fellow Austinites:

Even Woody Hayes occasionally had to say it, ... and now it is my turn to
say it -- "Punt!" But, the game isn't over yet.

As I leave The Austin Company, however, I want you to know that I feel
this change is both predestined and appropriate and bodes good for me in
the long run.

I want to thank each of you as appropriate for your loving-kindness,
compassion, support and assistance in the past, and particularly in the
last few months. Especially, I want those who worked with me most
closely to know that you will be remembered most warmly.

Thank you Austin Co. for 13, almost 14 years of scores of projects,
extensive travels throughout North America, and many, many rich and
varied memories ...

The torch is passed ... my run as an Austinite is over. To those who
continue on I say to take heart and "Go for it!" For life is in the
journey, the destination for each of us is at best uncertain.

As for my plans, they are crystalizing with surprising rapidity as my
second wind energizes me. When I renew my life's quest (which will be
shortly), it will probably be in another capacity in another city. As
surely as life as an honors student in a small high school in West
Virginia was followed by life as a struggling graduate student at Ohio
State; as surely as that was followed by a period of government
employment, life as a straw boss over a Puerto Rican maintenance crew in
the Islands, life as a cab driver in a small southern town, and life as a
consultant for The Austin Company, yet another "world" now beckons this
geographer's attentions.

Again, best wishes to each and every one of you in your separate lives
and to The Austin Company.

Sincerely yours,

Ronald F. Doyle
Senior Location Consultant (Ret.)
Facilities Location Department

RFD/jg

APPENDIX

WORK PERFORMED DESCRIBED...
(IN INTERFACE WITH ECONOMIC DEVELOPMENT)

HOW TO MARKET YOUR COMMUNITY
WITH A SITE LOCATION CONSULTANT

Marketing your community to location consultants involves three essential thrusts. The first of these is understanding the role of the location consultant in the overall location process. The second is responding to the (real) needs of the consultant. The third, and perhaps the most important of all, is being responsible in all that you do in presenting your community's qualifications as a location for business.

The Consultant's Role & The Location Process

When a company brings in a consultant or consulting firm to advise on the location of a planned corporate facility, chances are that locational preferences have already been explored by members of the corporate location decision-making team. Either deadlocks between the members have emerged, or feelings of inadequacy of time/expertise have surfaced as to how to more exactly quantify, qualify, and select the best location from among those available and/or being considered. A location decision for a new facility is one of the most important decisions affecting the success of a venture (whatever kind it is). It is also one that after the decision has been made, is usually the least easily corrected. Because of its gravity, the decision is made most often by the top corporate personnel. Depending upon the size of the company and frequency of location decision-making these people already have broad knowledge of operating conditions nationwide or regionally. They also likely have extensive general and technical knowledge, have succeeded in the climb up the corporate ladder into the positions they now (often tenuously) hold, and have the concomitant personal egos, talents, political acuities and/or insecurities associated with these positions. Often they're also behind schedule and, depending upon the corporate culture, need answers soon. It is into this atmosphere that the location consultant or consulting firm is brought . . .

If the first meeting is successful and the efforts of the consultant or consulting firm [1] have resulted in a contract to do location work, the next step is a careful gathering of the specific operating requirements of the facility to be located and a definition of the geographical and technical scope of work to be done. Once armed with this knowledge, the screening process busily begins.

---

[1] Austin works with a manager/staff consultant and support team concept. While the manager takes responsibility for the overall direction and implementation of the study, the location consultant is the project engineer who field investigates, processes in-office data and directs graphics/secretarial report preparation. The staff consultant himself consults with the manager and other associates brought in from the rest of the company to advise on various aspects of the location study at appropriate stages to obtain concurrence.

WORK PERFORMED DESCRIBED...
(IN INTERFACE WITH ECONOMIC DEVELOPMENT)

The Screening Process

There are three levels of screening that lead to targeting a specific site and community for the location of a project. These levels are national, regional and local. In the first instance, the consultant attempts to define what regions (areas) within the nation offer the best situation for his client. Then, within those regions, which communities are most favorable. Finally, within selected favorable communities, which sites maximize the client's location potential.

In the typical location study, the screening process involves narrowing down the list of all possible locations to a short list of locations which offer the most favorable operating conditions for the proposed operation. It is a negative elimination process in which all areas are given initially an equal chance at being selected and an extensive search is made to eliminate locations one-by-one which do not well meet the operating requirements of the facility. That resultant short list, depending upon the type of study, can be geographical regions or specific sites in an area. However, ultimately, screening involves defining a series of site/situation conditions within specific communities which most favor the successful operation of the proposed facility.

If the operation is a manufacturing plant, for example, preliminary data on freight costs, labor, utilities, taxes, and special facility requirements is gathered, and preferred status given to low cost/compatible locations. The location consultant field investigates those selected locations in order to update and expand upon his data base on them and gain first-hand current knowledge of operating conditions in these locations.

A careful analysis follows next whereby further screening of the field investigated locations yields the more highly favorable locations from among the others. These better locations are yet more thoroughly investigated and analyzed. At Austin, three (usually) are then determined to be "recommended" (i.e., those locations of all locations that appear to offer the least impediment to the success of the proposed operation). These recommended are then most rigorously investigated, depending upon time and budget constraints. Advantages and disadvantages are meticulously spelled out, and an intensive economic analysis is made.

An experienced manager and an informed location consultant together conclude a ranking of recommended communities and the locational recommendations. A client report and other communication materials are then prepared, and a presentation by the location consultant and the manager is made to the client decision-making team. Throughout this entire screening process, the location consultant (team) is the buyer's representative, the client's surrogate. For the duration, the location consulting team must think like him, and act only in his behalf, and be free of any intramural prejudices.

WORK PERFORMED DESCRIBED...
(IN INTERFACE WITH ECONOMIC DEVELOPMENT)

The Client Visit

An equally important phase of the location begins after the client has accepted the recommendations. Austin has always urged a visit to the recommended sites by the client's decision-making team. At this point, there is, ideally, a tentative modification in the role of the location consultant as the client's team assumes buyer beware posture. Depending upon the response of the client team to location inspection, the location consultant calibrates his own posture. If the client team tends toward the naive and overly trustful, the staff consultant reinstills buyer beware attitude in the client team. If the client team tends toward too much suspicion and negativity, the staff consultant will calibrate his posture to sell the advantages and elaborate on how to minimize the disadvantages of the locations recommended to the client team. Maintenance by the client of "arm's length" objectivity is absolutely necessary. But, a careful analysis has been made by the location firm already, and client "buying" of the recommendations for serious inquiry by their technical support people advances the whole project team toward meeting the project schedule.

Client Follow-Up

The final (determining) phase in the location selection process begins as client technical support teams thoroughly investigate the recommended locations, usually as an option to buy a site has been taken by the client (or by the consulting firm confidentially in the client's name).

Location consultants usually are generalists (they know something about just about everything but seldom have extreme depth of knowledge in every subject involved in a location decision) -- and that's fine in the initial stages of location. But now with a preliminary selection of a final location (or set of locations), technical expertise (specific) should be applied to discern detailed operating conditions in the areas of labor, transportation, utilities, construction, and other realms significant to the success of the venture. The client knows his own business location needs best Detailed site specific boundary surveys, test wells, core drillings, title searches, construction labor recruitment and organizational analysis, and building design adaptation/ cost reanalysis are made during this period by client personnel and technical subcontractors.

It is only after these matters are sufficiently checked in detail that a final corporate commitment to build is announced, and an option on land becomes an agreement to purchase the site. By this time also, the original location consultant has probably been reassigned to another project (his knowledge was limited vis-a-vis the experts; his knowledge is also becoming dated) and even the manager's role becomes minimal as squads of specialists have replaced the initial lone location consultant in the locale of the target site.

WORK PERFORMED DESCRIBED...
(IN INTERFACE WITH ECONOMIC DEVELOPMENT)

Responding To The Location Consultant's Needs

The greatest need of the location consultant is born of his generalist
background. It is not the need to be 100% right -- but the need to not
be wrong ... about anything that is said or written ... at each location.

There is usually time to fine-tune comprehension during the location
process (either at the consultant stage, the client visit, or during the
period of the option and client investigation); but wrong assessments,
wrong data at the early stages have multiplier effects down the line.
The consultant's initial visit is relatively inexpensive to the client
and community alike. The client's visit is more expensive (top salaries
are usually being paid to the decision-making team, and multiply this
times the duration of the visit and the number of visitors), as is the
community interface. And an option on property together with specialist
investigations and appropriate community response is more expensive yet.
The consultant needs to know as early as possible whether or not he is in
the wrong location -- and the consultant's inquiries are directed most
importantly toward this end.

The second need of the location consultant is to know how well the
location fits the client's facility's requirements, if it does. This
will be necessary to segregate the more favorable from the less favorable
locations, and in defining the degree of difference between locations (as
well as the overall magnitudes of project costs fine-tuned to specific
locations). The first information is needed to determine the recommended
locations, the second as input back to the client to determine if the
project itself is as feasible as the client originally thought it was
when he initiated the site search.

Concurrent to these two needs is, most often, the consultant's need for
client confidentiality. The confidentiality of consultant inquiries and
visits is required for several reasons:

1) Often clients seek to locate new facilities with as little
    advance warning to competitors as possible.

2) Often client facility searches, if known about in their home
    office (or existing operations), could spur inaccurate rumoring
    and undue panic among people who may not even be affected by
    whatever decision is made.

3) Site costs in communities under investigation could escalate with
    premature disclosure. (This happens and sometimes kills or relo-
    cates projects. Even though the land is a small part of the
    overall project cost -- all costs contribute to the bottom-line
    cost).

4) Some location searches are politically sensitive (for a host of
    reasons ranging from environmental to financial and/or regional
    economic reasons). Premature disclosure to "those who do not
    need to know yet" can trigger political actions on an inappro-
    priately large scale; killing or relocating projects that, were
    there time to develop the proper data for purposes of public

WORK PERFORMED DESCRIBED...
(IN INTERFACE WITH ECONOMIC DEVELOPMENT)

relations, should have gone forth -- and in so doing would have been of positive benefit to the selected community, its region, and/or the nation. (Other times, the client will deliberately trigger a political reaction to encourage inter-regional competition for his facility ... but that is his decision and timing to do so, not the location consultant's).

5)   There are also a myriad of other reasons.

Economic development representatives can greatly help enhance their community's chances for appropriate consideration by respecting and being responsive to the location consultant's (real) needs. Accurate information, honest reflective opinions from an economic development representative (especially an honest "I don't know -- if you don't know), and confidentiality enhance the possibilities that your location will receive proper attention.

Being Responsible

Be responsible in that which you do. Accuracy and completeness of information should be (if it isn't) a cardinal rule of economic development practice and community marketing. There are a few common situations that I have noticed in dealing with communities that need to be addressed -- these still often remain a significant problem to serving client needs:

Disinformation

An obvious quick-fix approach to economic development (particularly by a hungry community) is unfortunately still sometimes to "lie". Especially this is often done (if it will be done) to the location consultant in order to get a chance to "convince" the principals (client).

Blatant lies are getting rarer as the economic development world gets smarter in its own interests.

A more painful problem, however, sometimes occurs and with greater frequency than actual deceit. Inaccuracies (non-facts), especially those that are sincerely believed by the speakers of them, stand a better chance of getting through the location screening process than outright lies. There is no hesitation of voice, no diversion of the eyes -- not much to give it away at first. The unintentional error, if not caught, is sometimes passed right up the line and believed by everyone ultimately to be true.

It is a location consultant's job to attempt to ascertain the accuracy of the information given him, but often time constraints and study scope (number of locations considered) do not permit him to completely glean "the wheat from the chaff". (It is for this reason that the location process has several steps: the location consultant taking a short time at each of many locations to investigate everything; the client visit [several people taking a short time in a few places to reinvestigate everything]; and the option period [several people taking a long time at one or two locations to reinvestigate everything again]).

WORK PERFORMED DESCRIBED...
(IN INTERFACE WITH ECONOMIC DEVELOPMENT)

The important note here is that any community that misleads a consultant works against its own interests, too. A responsible development representative should be apprehensive about getting caught in a disinformation trap -- for the location process is very expensive to the client and community alike -- especially the further down the process it goes until the disinformation is exposed.

A responsible development official should be even more apprehensive, however, about untrue information not getting caught. A wrong location decision based on a "lie" not caught results in great expense for the client company forced to close (or downscale) its newly opened facility; a bad feeling among the community workforce hired, then laid off; an unhappy corporate community member until they leave; and often an empty building to be remarketed for the community.

The economic effects on the client (and his consultants) and the community (and their people) are that everybody suffers.

Most responsible community representatives do not encourage growth for growth's sake, but seeking the long-run interests of the community, seek those facilities that, in truth, can best operate from their locations successfully.

Statistics/Information Completeness

Completeness of information creates an additional problem area in facility location. Comparing apples with apples, that is, having similar-type/date data on all locations is often crucial to a good location decision. Sometimes comparable information is simply not available -- and the objectivity and, perhaps, accuracy of the analysis will suffer somewhat. But if the information is available, the community serves its own best interests by making such requested data available to the consultant, as well as to the client or client's support people in follow-up visits as requested.

Timeliness

At various stages of the location process, culling decisions have to be made to keep on schedule. Ninety percent (+) of facts needed to make a decision are usually readily available or quickly obtainable by a location consultant. That remaining 10% may, however, be crucial to correct decision making. Anything community marketers can do to get the remaining necessary information to the consultant in a timely fashion (short of compromising accuracy, that is) helps ensure continued consideration of the community in the site selection process.

The entire post screening effort of the location consultant team is directed toward the timely identification of problem areas (before they can detract from the success of a project), communicating them to the client, and posing (or getting the client to think about) remedies. That should also be the client decision-making team's focus, the focus of client technical and support experts, and the prime interest of the community promoters from the inception of the location process on into operations of the client facility on the selected location.

WORK PERFORMED DESCRIBED...
(IN INTERFACE WITH ECONOMIC DEVELOPMENT)

Albeit, even with a multi-lateral enthusiastic commitment to timely accuracy and completeness of information, no perfect location is ever found -- for there are none. Also, "The best laid plans of mice and men sometimes go awry ..." as sometimes the pressure of genuine time constraints coupled with less than optimal communication can also detract from a project's success potential.

But honest, accurate, and complete information transmitted in a timely fashion should minimize the numbers of and damage sustained in these occasional location mishaps.

In summary, marketing your community with location consultants involves three simple steps that, if properly and meticulously executed, can't help but have positive long-term pay-backs for the community, the locating firms, the consulting engineers, and ultimately for the community representatives, too. They are:

1) Understand the location process.

2) Be responsive to it at each step; and

3) Be responsible in all that you do.

These steps are most often best initiated simultaneously or in tandem, and are admittedly much easier said than done. However, the degree of their implementation will determine the degree of long-term success of your community marketing program with location consultants as well as with their principals (clients).

THIS IS TO CERTIFY THAT

Ronald F. Doyle

being qualified and having subscribed to

the Council's Members' Code as engrossed below, has been

elected to membership in the

American Industrial Development Council

MEMBERS' CODE

Know all men by these presents that members of the Council are dedicated to:

Maintain the highest ethical standards in professional relationships.

Advance the best civic and economic interests of the communities and areas served.

Uphold the dignity and prestige associated with Council membership.

Cooperate with fellow members in informal exchange of
information and ideas reflecting practices, procedures, trends, and policy
pertaining to industrial development.

Accept personal responsibility for furthering the
Council's program when called upon.

In testimony whereof witness the signatures of the officers of the Council

This *15th* day of *February, 1979*

Robert E. Leak
PRESIDENT

Barbara Clements
Acting EXECUTIVE VICE PRESIDENT

MEANWHILE AT THE OFFICE AND IN THE FIELD . . .
PROJECT NOTES AND HIGHLIGHTS (1973-1976)

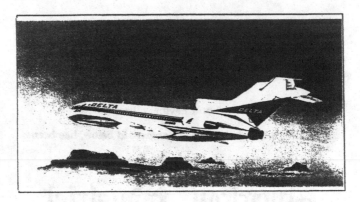

FIRST . . .

A couple of favorable area studies were done in the office under direct supervision. The first study lasted a few weeks. I never met the client.

NEXT . . .

The second study was also done in the office. It also lasted a few weeks. I talked to the client briefly over the telephone on the results.

NEXT . . .
A SITE STUDY (1974)

I worked (in training) with another staff consultant on this project. My part was done first in the office, then later on a site search in the field in San Antonio, Texas in which I participated. This plant was eventually located in San Antonio and operated there. My part of the study lasted a few weeks. For my part, I became familiar with the San Antonio area of that era.

NEXT . . .
CLARK EQUIPMENT COMPANY (1974)

This was my first major locational assignment. It was a study and analysis for three of Clark's divisions: Melroe (bobcat) division, construction machinery division; and, the fork lift division. There was extensive in office and in the field work. Field studies took me to several Alabama communities including Huntsville; several communities in Georgia and North Carolina. Working for my management, I also coordinated with the client's real estate department, principally at Clark.

HIGHLIGHTS: Clark's real estate man and I were attacked by hornets while inspecting a site in Trov, Alabama . . . but, I escaped unscathed! He and I were also both offered what sounded like a bribe by a local development official (a delivered side of beef) . . . We both reported thus: up our individual lines to management (as a matter of ethics). I coordinated a site tour (by the top Clark officials) by telephone keeping their identity secret. However, local ID (industrial development) later reported to me that they knew who it was because one of the top officers carried a CLARK briefcase and they had checked at the airport the registration on Clarks private plane used on the tour.

RESULTS: Austin was double-teamed on this project by the client's other location consultants. Their construction machinery plant eventually went to Asheville, North Carolina; their forklift plant to Rockingham, North Carolina; and, their bobcat division to Huntsville, Alabama.

PERSONAL (NON-MONETARY) GAIN: Familiarity with operating conditions in several area of "Dixie' in the era. Contact with Governor Wallace's economic development department through a Vietnam veteran with whom I established a business-related rapport back then.

NEXT . . .
TOTINO'S FINER FOODS (1974)

This was a favorable area and community/site study for their frozen pizza operation. My part lasted several months and involved in office analyses and field studies of many Tennessee/Kentucky area communities. Working under Bob Will I interfaced with Totino's board of plant location decision makers in Minnesota on several occasions. Ultimately their people decided on the site I had recommended in Murfreesboro, Tennessee. The plant was built there—Bob Will having concluded the option on the property covertly for Totino's working with local ID people.

HIGHLIGHTS: I visited about a dozen communities on this tour and worked with their ID reps. In Murfreesboro, I worked with the local judge, an impressive (conservative democrat) local powerhouse in his own right. During the site tour of Murfreesboro, the former ROTC commander at OSU got in the car at one point—he was living there then. We chatted about old times at OSU—good times and bad.

RESULTS: Totino's built with Austin on the site selected by me at Murfreesboro. For the first time, I had helped 'make a difference' on a location study.

PERSONAL GAIN: Seeing a small town judge in action made my job a lot easier. He was very dedicated and I felt good about this community because of him.

A METROPOLITAN NEWSPAPER (1975)

This was a site study for a satellite newspaper publishing plant. Most of my part I did in the field in Contra Costa and Alemeda Counties (San Francisco Bay Area) with a write-up in the office. The study took a couple of months. At the end, as at the beginning, I met with the client's rep at their city offices.

HIGHLIGHTS: I found myself muddling through great confusion as California's environmental and other laws seemed quite different and more complicated than in other parts of the country, and economic development assistance was, at the time, less. But, the job got done. A site in San Ramon was first recommended.

RESULTS: Recommendations were never acted on . . . The client decided if he expands it will be on his existing property in the city.

PERSONAL GAIN: Familiarity with the diversity and charm of the San Francisco Bay Area (a favorite part of the USA for me in that era). Several weekends—free time there—were paid for by The Austin Company (in lieu of the costs of flying me home and back on the weekends).

NEXT . . .
OWATONNA TOOL (1975)

This was a favorable area study lasting for a few weeks and done at the Cleveland office. No action resulted at that time.

NEXT . . .
AKRON CLIENT (1975)

This was a site study for an equipment manufacturer in the Greater Akron (Ohio) area. After several weeks of study in the field, I recommended a site at Stow. No action was ever taken that I know of.

HIGHLIGHT: The company president upon seeing the recommended site, gleefully leaped from the site tour car I was driving and onto the site at Stow—in enthusiasm to get his project started! But, as I said, despite his pleased enthusiasm, I am not aware of any action ever taken.

NEXT . . .
AMOCO REALTY (1975)

This was a study of multiple sites for an environmentally objectionable acid plant. I checked out one site and another staff consultant checked out the others. We compared notes. The report was then submitted to the client.

HIGHLIGHT: I met the site owners' rep at Charleston, South Carolina Airport and rode with him aboard his small plane to Myrtle Beach. There we transferred first to his car, then to his boat, then to his jeep to get to the interior of the 2000 acre site (Great Sandy Island). We explored it by vehicle and on foot, each section. Then, we returned by nightfall.

RESULTS: After comparative analysis, that particular site was not recommended for this project.

PERSONAL GAIN: A brief adventure.

NEXT . . .
NISSIN FOODS (1976)

This was a favorable area and site/community study for the location of an oriental noodle manufacturing plant. My part took about two to three months. The first part was done in the office.

For the second part, 1 travelled to several Maryland and Eastern Pennsylvania communities, focusing on Pennsylvania Dutch country, making community, labor/site studies.

HIGHLIGHT: Dinner at a farm house, Pennsylvania Dutch style. After visiting the client to make a report, I also later played poker at a poker palace in Gardena, California.

RESULTS: The client, a California based Japanese firm, chose a recommended site in Lancaster, Pennsylvania and built his plant there.

PERSONAL GAIN: Travel to California to meet the client . . . also I toured Disneyland while I was there; a thorough visit to Pennsylvania Dutch country.

NEXT . . .
A COFFEE PROCESSOR (1976)

This was a favorable area and a site/community study for a coffee, processing plant. The first part took about a month or two. For the second part, I travelled to New Orleans, Louisiana, Gulfport-Biloxi, Mississippi, and Pensacola, Florida.

HIGHLIGHT: A weekend (company paid) in the French Quarter of New Orleans; dinner at Antoine's and several other restaurants.

RESULTS: No action was ever taken on this project.

PERSONAL GAIN: Travel to west coast (for a client meeting); pleasant trips to communities, a "hurricane" drink at O'Brien's, and an evening at Preservation Hall Dixieland Hall in the French Quarter.

NEXT . . .
ANOTHER FAVORABLE AREA DETERMINATION (1976)

This was an in-office study of short duration. No action was taken on this project that I was aware of.

NEXT . . .
ATS / EASTERN DISTRICT (1976)

This was a massive site search of the New Jersey section of the Greater Metropolitan NYC Area accomplished by myself and a teammate staff consultant. It was to find a location (or locations) for two of Austin's own divisions: Eastern District (construction) and ATS (military weapons systems).M y part took about two months or so. I studied the area north of the Raritan to the New York border and west to Dover, travelling extensively therein.

HIGHLIGHT: Visits with family then in the area nearby. Visit to my Amelia Avenue house (my childhood home).

RESULTS: Austin located each division on sites in that area. The study identified many considerations.

PERSONAL GAIN: Refamiliarization with my childhood surroundings, the changes since, and the scope and breadth of the NYC area. It seemed to me to be a hard area to get much done in a timely fashion compared to other areas of the country.

NOTE: After this study, Bob Will became head of the entire Technical Services Division at Austin Headquarters and Steve Appleby became facilities location manager.

EVALUATIONS

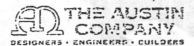

THE AUSTIN COMPANY
DESIGNERS · ENGINEERS · BUILDERS

DEPARTMENT CORRESPONDENCE
PLEASE REPLY ON ATTACHED SHEET

TO __R. A. Hill__   FROM __S. R. A__

OFFICE OR JOB __Technical Services__   RETURN THIS TO OFFICE OR JOB __Technical Services__

SUBJECT: Employee Performance and Compensation   DATE __February 9, 1978__
Ronald F. Doyle

As part of our continuing evaluation of employee performance and compensation, this memorandum is intended to provide information for the employee's personnel file to be used in the review process.

I have been especially well pleased with Ron's work attitude and performance since the start of my assignment. He has been, by far, the most productive and dedicated member of our department. He has shown continuous and significant improvement in developing recommendations, writing reports, and relating to the Clients. I believe he deserves significant compensation consideration on a merit basis for his contribution to our departmental efforts.

I will work with Ron to continue to improve his analytical abilities and his Client presentation efforts. I am confident that he will continue to be a very valuable asset to our department and company.

SRA/jm

cc: T. B. Sweeney
    S. G. Richardson

MEANWHILE AT THE OFFICE AND IN THE FIELD . . .
PROJECT NOTES AND HIGHLIGHTS: 1976-1984
(while working under S. R. Appleby)

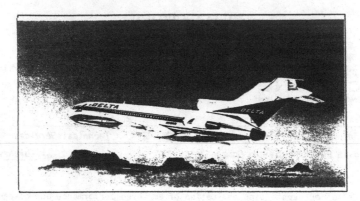

NEXT . . .
A MANUFACTURING CO. (1977)

This was a favorable area study done mostly in the office. Study results were presented to the Client in their Memphis office a few weeks after starting the study. No actions resulted.

NEXT . . .
ECKERD DRUG (1977)

This was a site study in the southwestern part of the metropolitan Atlanta area. My part took a month or so. I enjoyed the hospitality of some of the ED and real estate people who helped me during the project (excellent Southern-style eating at exclusive area restaurants). An Eckerd drug distribution center was, I believe, later established on one of the recommended sites.

NEXT . . .
COMMERCIAL PRESS DIV., HARRIS CORP. (1978)

This was a metropolitan labor study of the Greater DFW (Dallas-Ft. Worth) area. My part took a month or so of in-the-field work plus write-up time. I coordinated on the project with my management and a representative of Harris Corp., who regularly debriefed me as I went along with the study.

HIGHLIGHT: Taking Harris' CEO (Boyd) on a tour of the DFW area with his assistants and my manager.

RESULTS: Harris Corp. transferred its commercial press operation to DFW onto a site near the DFW Airport.

PERSONAL GAIN: Travel, familiarity with the DFW area of that era.

NEXT . . .
OWATONNA TOOL (1978)

This was a favorable area and community/site study to locate a branch plant for this company's expanding product line of tools for automobiles. My part took 2 to 4 months. After in-office work, I travelled to a dozen communities in the Kentucky/Tennessee/Arkansas favorable area.

HIGHLIGHT: Thanks to cooperation from the recommended communities, a successful site tour was concluded allowing the Kaplan brothers, Owatonna Tools owners, to get a good overview of the competing locations quickly.

RESULT: A recommended location in Searcy, AR was selected by OTC. Austin built the plant.

PERSONAL GAIN: Satisfaction that a client was satisfied.

NEXT . . .
MIDLAND-ROSS GRIMES DIV.

This was a site study in Urbana, Ohio. Of short duration, several locations were selected, one was chosen by Grimes, and they built their new facility on it.

PERSONAL GAIN: This was a pleasant experience working in western Ohio truly "God is in His heaven, and all is well with the world".

NEXT . . .

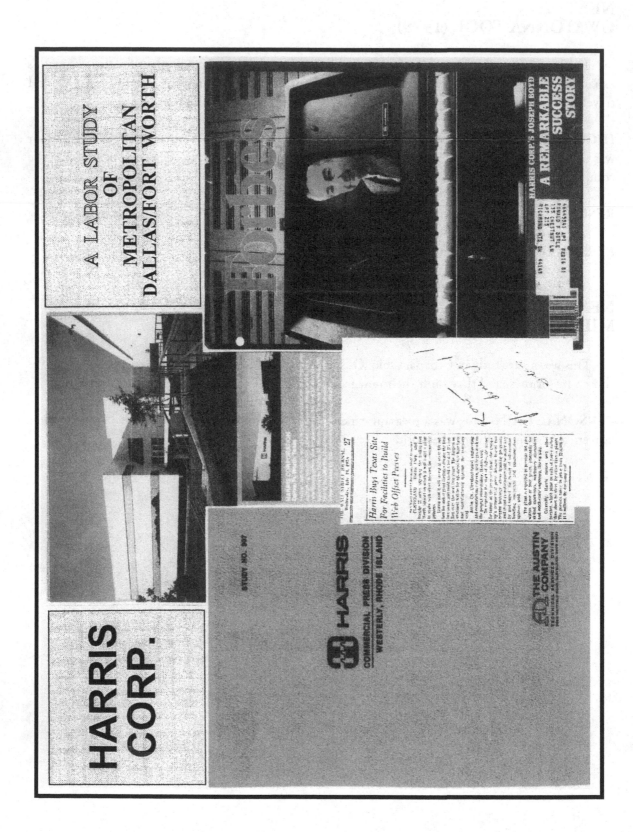

OWATONNA
TOOL
COMPANY

A FAVORABLE AREA
AND
COMMUNITY/SITE STUDY
IN
KENTUCKY, TENNESSEE
AND ARKANSAS

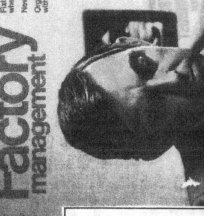

Factory management

May 1977

Fixtures: putting light where it does most good

New compressors debut

Organizing to comply with the regulations

Man of the Year

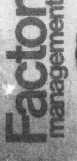
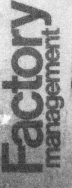
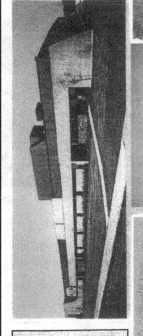

STUDY NUMBER 112

OWATONNA TOOL COMPANY
OWATONNA, MINNESOTA

OWATONNA TOOL COMPANY
Searcy, Arkansas

Owatonna is a familiar name among workshop owners and automotive tool users. When demand for its tools outgrew the company's production capabilities in Owatonna, Minnesota, Austin was commissioned to conceive and design a new plant, find a site for its location, and provide interior designs and furnishings for the office building that would serve the production facility.

Austin's Facilities Location group selected Searcy, Arkansas—some fifty miles northeast of Little Rock—in part because of its more central location to Owatonna's markets and material sources, and also for its potential operating cost reduction. Austin's Central District office provided the basic concept for the plant, did the detailed engineering drawings and prepared specifications, then supervised the construction of the plant and office. The selection, purchase and installation of the office furniture was also an Austin responsibility.

The 100,000-square-foot facility is framed with structural steel and sheathed with metal and precast architectural concrete panels. The distinctive design of the building facade was selected for an "Excellency in Concrete" award by the Arkansas Ready Mix Concrete Association.

THE AUSTIN COMPANY

DESIGNERS
ENGINEERS
BUILDERS

THE AUSTIN COMPANY
TECHNICAL SERVICES DIVISION

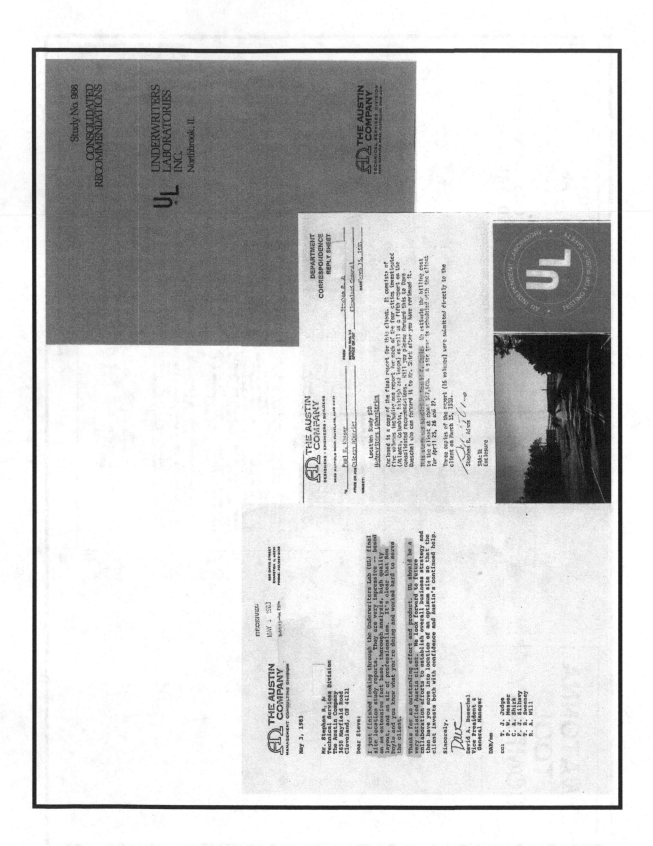

A CHEMICAL PLANT (1978)

This was a favorable area/community/site study for a chemical plant in the Carolinas. It took me a few months to do my part and involved much travel within North and South Carolina. Nothing much came of this project—nor do I think a plant was ever built

NEXT . . .
OLINKRAFT (1979)

This was a favorable area site and community study with also a metropolitan site study of the Los Angeles, Phoenix, and Las Vegas areas for a soft drink and beer carrier facility. Aside from spending several weeks in the Los Angeles to San Bernadino area, with side studies in the Greater Phoenix and Las Vegas-Henderson areas, I visited several smaller communities in Arizona and California, including Bakersfield. The whole study including presentations at West Monroe, Louisiana, and Cincinnati, Ohio, took several months.

HIGHLIGHTS: A good rapport was established with this client and I went along on several junkets of wining and dining their top people. A "grand tour" of the West afforded by this study was also impressively memorable, particularly a stay in Palm Springs, and a weekend on the Queen Mary. A drive down Red Oak Canyon produced some topographical photographs I treasure.

RESULTS: The client built on our recommended site in Bakersfield. They were pleased with our FLD work. However, another contractor got the construction award.

PERSONAL GAIN: Satisfaction that a client was pleased. Travel memories.

NEXT . . .
MYOJO FOODS (1979)

This was a favorable area and community/site study. Aside from work at the office, I spent a couple of weeks in the field assessing several Ohio/Indiana/Kentucky towns for the facility. The study in total took a couple of months and concluded with a site community tour led by myself and accompanied by several Japanese Myojo representatives.

HIGHLIGHTS: Dinner at Lebanon's Golden Lamb with the entire Japanese delegation.

RESULTS: Myojo located at Sidney, Ohio; Austin built the plant. (But, they never opened—their product did not market well in America. The facility, I understand, was later sold at a distressed price.)

PERSONAL GAIN: The project was successful from a location study standpoint.

NEXT . . .
A PRODUCTS PLANT (1980)

This was a favorable area study; it took six to eight weeks in the office. We met with the client in Chicago. No further action was taken.

NEXT . . .

OLINKRAFT

A COMMUNITY/SITE STUDY IN SOUTHERN CALIFORNIA, NEVADA, AND ARIZONA AND A SITE STUDY OF GREATER LOS ANGELES

KERN COUNTY ON THE MOVE!
Olinkraft to Build $16 Million Plant

Johns-Manville Corp.
Unit Will Build Plant

Study Number 927

OLINKRAFT
West Monroe, Louisiana

THE AUSTIN COMPANY

RECEIVED
AUG 09 1979

OLINKRAFT

August 7, 1979

FRED R. WEBB
Project Manager
Multiple Packaging

The Austin Company
Facilities Location Department
3650 Mayfield Road
Cleveland, Ohio 44121

Attention: Mr. Stephen R. Adams, Manager

Subject: Olinkraft Location Study 927 and 927-A

Dear Steve:

This is to advise that the final report for the subject location study has been reviewed and found acceptable by our personnel. With this acceptance, all work under the applicable purchase order for this study is considered to be complete. Final invoices should be submitted at the earliest possible date.

As you know by now from our prior conversations, we have selected and are pursuing the recommended site in the City of Bakersfield, California.

Sincerely,

Fred R. Webb
Project Manager
Multiple Packaging Division   OLINKRAFT, Inc.

My best experience...

AN ELECTRIC CO (1980) (1983)

These were a series of favorable area and site community studies done to assess appropriate locations for the client's weapons systems facilities including the TUA weapons system and the electronic warfare division plant of Emerson Electric Co. They involved together many months of work and in the field (lower profile) investigations particularly in Texas but also in several other southern states.

HIGHLIGHT: Interesting company-sponsored tour of the Greenville to San Antonio electronics corridor and plants with 'star wars' technology.

RESULTS: No follow-up information on what the client decided was ever given me—nor did I inquire.

PERSONAL GAIN: The jobs helped some—I later saw pictures of the TUA weapons system shown in a National Guard publication.

NEXT . . .
TRW (1980)

This was a favorable area and site/community study done to find a location for a jet engines mold plant. It involved me in studying in the field several communities in the Carolinas and Virginia.

HIGHLIGHT: In North Carolina, I met with a number of interested citizens including the former governor, Terry Sanford.

RESULTS: TRW located and built their plant on the recommended site in Sanford, NC.

PERSONAL GAIN: General satisfaction with this location project by most.

NEXT . . .
KHK (BIOKYOWA): 1981

This was a favorable area and site/community study of Illinois, Missouri, Tennessee and Kentucky for the location of a Japanese amino acid additive plant (cattle feed additive). The locational requirements of this facility were extremely complex and I needed and received much assistance from local development people. I visited several communities intensively studying the possibilities offered by many large sites screened and selected. The study from start to finish took several months and concluded with a site tour led by myself and including a significant Japanese delegation from KHK.

HIGHLIGHT: The site tour went well as I and the Process Division assistant manager entertained and were entertained by the KHK group as we toured together recommended sites in Kansas City, St. Louis, and Cape Girardeau.

RESULTS: The client built a large facility on the site in the back-up community of Cape Girardeau. Several things went wrong with this project, however, and I personally received some deserved and some undeserved negative exposure before my management.

PERSONAL GAIN: I learned to mute more my positive comments in response to allegations of 'overselling'. (NOTE: Staff consultants got no reward for steering a client to any particular site or town. I had no motive to oversell) I hurt all over for a long time. My career began its downward slide. But, I was allowed to keep my job.

NEXT . . .
ANOTHER JAPANESE CLIENT (1981)

This was a favorable area study that took a few weeks of in office work, was reviewed at Cleveland by a large Japanese delegation and resulted in nothing further.

NEXT . . .
COPPERWELD TUBING GROUP (1981)

This was an extensive study involving both community and site analyses. It included several metropolitan site studies done in western Tennessee, Arkansas, Oklahoma, Louisiana and Texas (Houston area). It was for an oil field tubing plant. Extensive field studies kept me travelling and making reports most of the year. In the end, the project was cancelled as the oil boom ended and Copperweld was itself seized by the French government.

HIGHLIGHTS: Lunch at Suzette's in Little Rock as Steve and I listened to the problems Phillipe Rothschild was having with the Mitterand government as relayed to us by the Copperweld's dutifully over concerned owner's rep. We Austinites, both of lower middle class background now sampling foods we both had only previously read about, exuded tears of sympathy when we realized 'into every man's life some rain must fall,' even a Rothchild's.

RESULTS: Nothing happened. The project was shelved.

PERSONAL GAIN: A saga concluded.

NEXT . . .

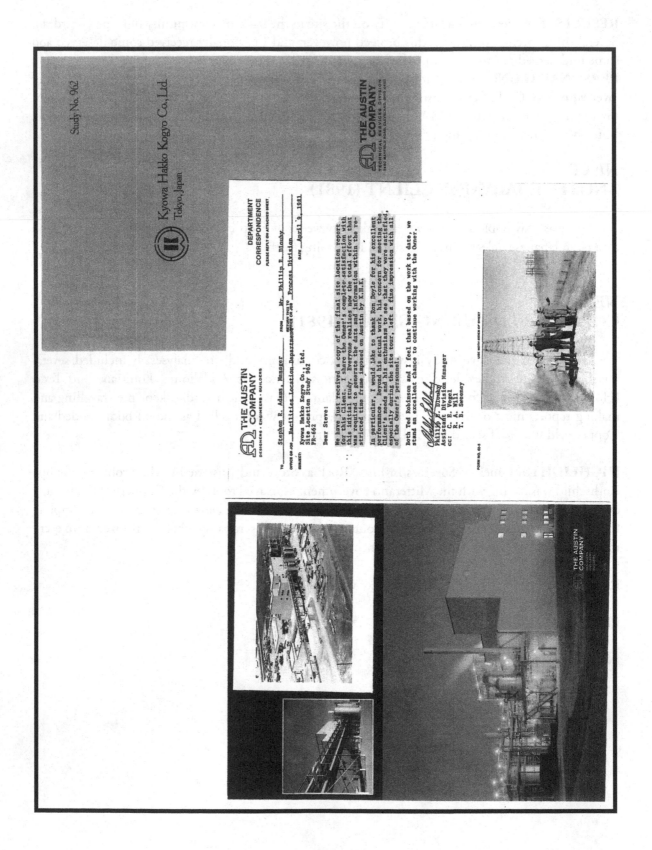

Study No. 962

Kyowa Hakko Kogyo Co., Ltd
Tokyo, Japan

THE AUSTIN COMPANY
TECHNICAL SERVICES DIVISION
3650 MAYFIELD ROAD, CLEVELAND, OHIO 44121

THE AUSTIN COMPANY
DESIGNERS · ENGINEERS · BUILDERS

DEPARTMENT
CORRESPONDENCE
PLEASE REPLY ON ATTACHED SHEET.

TO Stephen R. Adams, Manager FROM Mr. Phillip F. Dlouhy
     Facilities Location Department   RETURN THIS TO Process Division
                                      OFFICE OR JOB
                                      DATE April 9, 1981

OFFICE OR JOB

SUBJECT: Kyowa Hakko Kogyo Co., Ltd.
         Site Location Study 962
         PR-662

Dear Steve:

We have just received a copy of the final site location report
for this Client. I share the Owner's complete satisfaction with
this initial study. Everyone realizes now the total effort that
was required to generate the data and information within the re-
stricted time frame imposed on Austin by K.H.K.

In particular, I would like to thank Ron Doyle for his excellent
performance. Beyond his actual work, his concern for meeting the
Client's needs and his enthusiasm to see that they were satisfied,
especially during the site tour, left a fine impression with all
of the Owner's personnel.

Both Ted Robinson and I feel that based on the work to date, we
stand an excellent chance to continue working with the Owner.

Phillip F. Dlouhy
Assistant Division Manager
cc: C. E. Vogel
    R. A. Mill
    T. B. Sweeney

FORM NO. 63-3

THE AUSTIN COMPANY

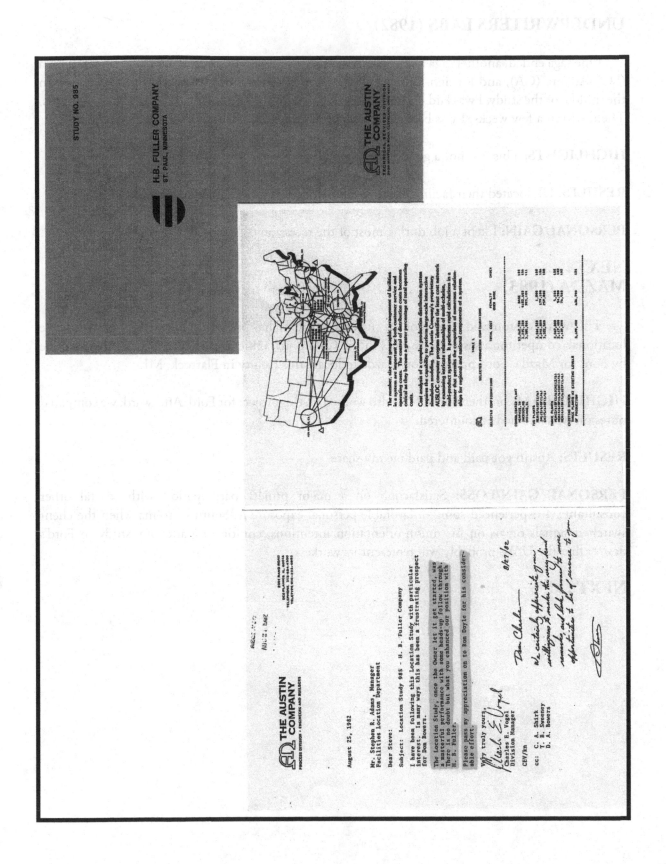

UNDERWRITERS LABS (1982)

One saga ended, another saga began: this was a metropolitan site study of Tampa (FL), Columbia (SC), Atlanta (GA), and Raleigh-Durham (NC), for the location of UL's southeastern facilities. In the middle of the study, I was laid off from work due to national and corporate economic conditions. Then, within a few weeks, I was brought back on full time and finished the study.

HIGHLIGHTS: This was not a good time in my life.

RESULTS: UL located their facility in the recommended Research Triangle Park (NC).

PERSONAL GAIN: I kept a job during most of the recession of '82.

NEXT . . .
MAZDA (1983)

This was a customized metropolitan site study of Omaha, NE, and Greenville, SC with some locational 'competitor assessment' studies in the Columbus, Ohio area to interface with work done by Ford for Mazda. Ford prevailed on Mazda to locate this facility in Flatrock, MI.

HIGHLIGHT: My brother Tim at Ford also worked on this project for Ford. Afterward, we compared notes on what we had encountered.

RESULTS: Austin got paid and paid me my share.

PERSONAL GAIN/LOSS: Satisfaction on a major project participation with several other consultants. I experienced some unfavorable personal exposure in South Carolina when the client switched signals on us on his union orientation intentions, conforming after my study to Ford's desires that the UAW probably will represent its workers.

NEXT . . .

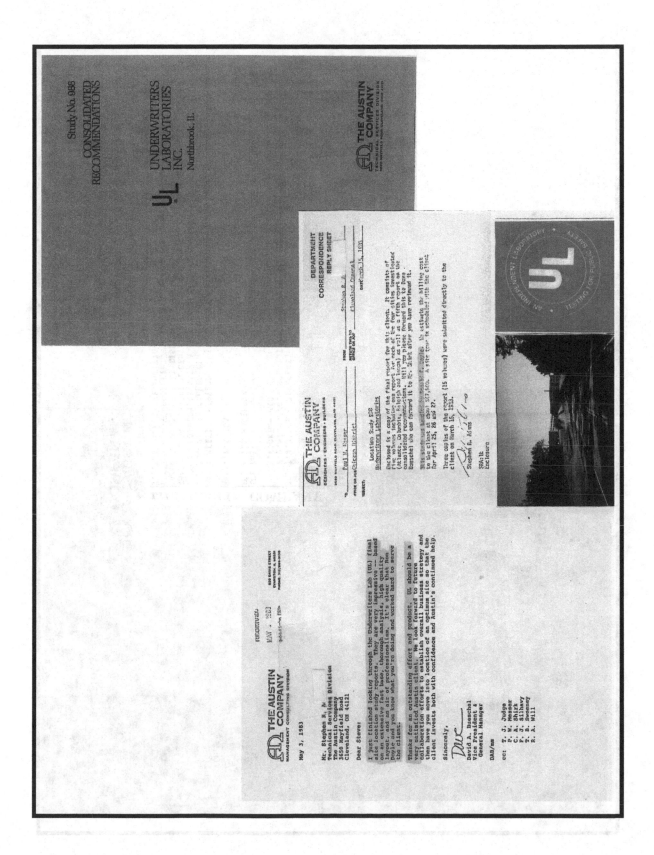

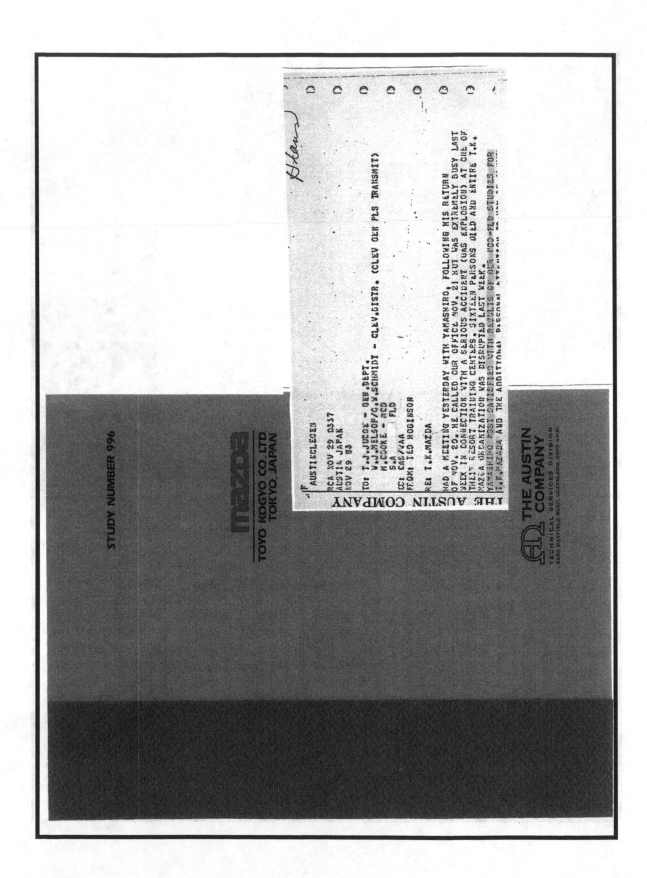

STUDY NUMBER 996

mazda

TOYO KOGYO CO. LTD.
TOKYO, JAPAN

THE AUSTIN COMPANY

THE AUSTIN COMPANY
TECHNICAL SERVICES DIVISION
3650 MAYFIELD ROAD CLEVELAND, OHIO 44121

AUSTINCLEGEM

RCA NOV 29 0337
AUSTIN JAPAN
NOV 29 83

TO: T.J.JUDGE - GEN.DEPT.
W.J.MELSOPPG,W.SCHMIDT - CLEV.DISTR. (CLEV GEN PLS TRANSMIT)
M.COONE - MCD
S.A - FLD
CC: CAS/YAA
FROM: TED ROBINSON

RE: T.K.MAZDA

HAD A MEETING YESTERDAY WITH YAMASHIRO, FOLLOWING HIS RETURN
OF NOV. 20. HE CALLED OUR OFFICE NOV. 21 BUT WAS EXTREMELY BUSY LAST
WEEK IN CONNECTION WITH A SERIOUS ACCIDENT (GAS EXPLOSION) AT ONE OF
THEIR RESORT TRAINING CENTERS. SIXTEEN PERSONS DIED AND ENTIRE T.K.
MAZDA ORGANIZATION WAS DISRUPTED LAST WEEK.
YAMASHIRO MOST SATISFIED WITH RESULTS OF OUR MCD-FLD STUDIES FOR
T.K.MAZDA AND THE ADDITIONAL PERSONAL ATTENTION TO HIS CONCERNS

A JAPANESE ELECTRIC CO (1983)

This was a favorable area study taking a few weeks and resulting in nothing afterwards.

NEXT . . .
ARVIN AUTOMOTIVE (1984)

This was a favorable area and site community study of Kentucky/Tennessee selected communities for a muffler plant.

HIGHLIGHT: The site tour with Arvin management went well.

RESULT: The client adapted an existing facility for his new operation.

PERSONAL GAIN: A pleasant tour of Columbus, IN, and many architecturally proper buildings there.

NEXT . . .
"BIG BROADCASTERS" OF NEW YORK (1984)

This was an alternative site study in Manhattan, other NYC boroughs, and the New Jersey Meadowlands for possible relocation of the headquarters of a large national communications company.

HIGHLIGHT: Dinner at The Russian Tea Room with my boss—Good thing caviar is not habit-forming. Several walking tours of Manhattan while there for several weeks by myself.

RESULTS: The report was well received, but nothing happened as a result of it that I was ever informed about.

PERSONAL GAIN: I bought a Salvador Dali print which became my prize treasure (then).

NOTE: Jim Broughton became manager as Steve Appleby was transferred to National Gypsum, our new owner. I had been passed over. But, in retrospect, they had made the right decision . . . my mind had been strained . . .

Study Number 1005
(text and tables only)

Arvin Automotive
Columbus, Indiana

THE AUSTIN COMPANY
DESIGNERS · ENGINEERS · BUILDERS

1205 FIFTH & RACE TOWER
CINCINNATI, OHIO 45202
TELEPHONE: 513/651-3585

RECEIVED
APR 30 1984
Technical Services Division

THE AUSTIN COMPANY
TECHNICAL SERVICES DIVISION
3650 MAYFIELD ROAD, CLEVELAND, OHIO 44121

April 26, 1984

Mr. Stephen A.
The Austin Company
3650 Mayfield Road
Cleveland, Ohio 44121

Dear Steve,

Just a word of thanks for the fine job you and your group recently
completed for Arvin Automotive in Columbus, Indiana. Ron Doyle, in
particular, deserves special recognition for a most professional
report, and for coordinating a very complicated community tour.

The Client has on several occasions, expressed his complete satis-
faction, and proven his confidence in Austin by releasing the
Cleveland District on a significant preliminary engineering effort.
There is every indication that a major construction release will
follow, and the opportunity is a direct result of a thorough Facility
Location Report.

I look forward to working with you again. Thanks, and well done!

Sincerely,

Jeffrey C. Pomeroy
Resident Manager

JCP/jb

MEANWHILE AT THE OFFICE AND IN THE FIELD . . .

PROJECT NOTES AND HIGHLIGHTS: 1984-1987

(while working under J. R. Boone)

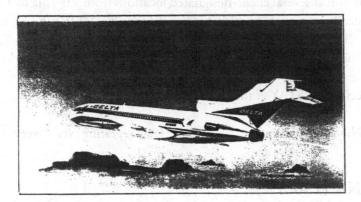

NEXT . . .
NATIONAL WATERLIFT (1984)

This was a community/site and strategic array study for an electronics and missile parts production facility. It involved my personal travel to several communities in many southern states, with decision-maker meetings in Kalamazoo and Boston.

HIGHLIGHT: I chauffeured a former four star general (WWII retired) around on one of the site tours. I also took a weekend later to visit the Boston area.

RESULTS: A plant was eventually located by the client in a community recommended in a parallel study.

PERSONAL GAIN: A favorable perspective on the defense industry expanded.

NEXT . . .
AUSTIN CO. (INTERNAL PLANNING) (1985)

This was an in-office analysis to determine an order of facility closings in the event of corporate contraction. My part took a couple of months. Then my further participation was cancelled as these duties and others were transferred to an outside consulting firm who was to do a study of the whole of Austin management practices to renew the firm itself.

(At this point I spent some time recuperating from a 'breakdown' and was hospitalized in February 1985).

CAST IRON (1985)

This was a brief study for a foundry operation. A few communities in Tennessee were visited and presentations made at Dayton. Nothing notable happened in result though. My part was praised by my co-consultant on this project.

NORTH CORP. (1985)

This study involved me checking in the field site/community suitability for a truck clutch manufacturing operation at several client-designated locations from Virginia to Tomalipas in Mexico. The project was basically to get information for the client's own MOVE/STAY decision-makers.

HIGHLIGHT: A study of conditions of operating at the Loredo-Nuevo Loredo border area.

RESULTS: They decided to STAY at their existing location.

PERSONAL GAIN: Travel/adventure . . . But, I was getting very, very tired of travel and adventure!

BARNETT BANK (1986)

This was a study to locate a bank data processing center in the St. Petersburg (Florida) area.

HIGHLIGHT: Exploring St. Petersburg as a hurricane loomed just offshore . . . and threatened to move in. (It didn't, however. A day later it began moving northwestward.)

RESULTS: The center was located.

PERSONAL GAIN: Some pleasant conversations with site owners over real estate and ED people.

AP de MEXICO (1986)

This was a brief project to double check for ARVIN (the owner) the decision of an AP de Mexico manager to move his muffler plant from Mexico City to another location in the Valley of Quereteros further north.

HIGHLIGHT: The local Austin manager, acted as chauffeur and interpreter. Because of him, I was able to complete my analysis of Mexico City, Quereteros, and another town considered, Toluca, efficiently. This is one of the few studies where I had regular company in the performance of my work.

RESULTS: I understand the plant was relocated to Quereteros in concurrence with the recommendations of the study.

PERSONAL GAIN: Greater familiarity with the diversity of Mexico, a third world country.

NEXT . . .
KONISHTROKU (1986)

My part was a site study in the Burlington/Greensboro part of North Carolina. The client eventually bought the recommended site and built on it. It was a two to three week study on my part, following up another consultant's work.

NEXT . . .
ARVIN-SANGO (1986)

This was a favorable area and site/community study for a joint venture muffler plant of Arvin Industries (Columbus, Indiana) and SANGO (Japan). The study took me to field visits to several communities in Indiana, Kentucky, and Ohio. It lasted a couple of months and concluded with a site tour with the client's personnel.

HIGHLIGHT: The site tour was successful.

RESULTS: The client located and built its facility in the recommended community of Madison, Indiana.

PERSONAL GAIN: Satisfaction. (But, this was to be my last major field study . . . I was simply wearing down again.)

NEXT . . .

AUSTIN UPDATE

MAY 1987

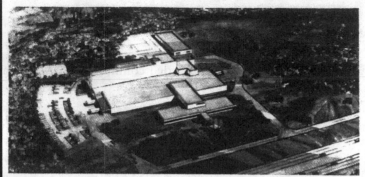

This photographic products plant is being designed and built for Konica Manufacturing U.S.A. in Greensboro, North Carolina, by a joint venture of The Austin Company and Shimizu America Corporation.

AUSTIN BEGINS CONSTRUCTION OF KONICA'S FIRST U.S. MANUFACTURING FACILITY

Konishiroku Photo Industries Co. Ltd., a leading Japanese manufacturer of photographic film, cameras, plain-paper copiers and floppy discs, has begun construction of a plant near Greensboro, North Carolina, its first in the United States.

The plant, which will be operated by a subsidiary, Konica Manufacturing U.S.A. Inc., is being designed to produce a variety of products, but initially will make photographic color paper.

The 84-acre site for the plant was selected after a study was conducted by the Facilities Location Department of The Austin Company.

Design, engineering and construction for the Konica facility are being performed by a joint venture of The Austin Company and Shimizu America Corporation.

Construction of the 300,000-square-foot facility will take approximately two years. The first manufacturing stage is scheduled to be on-line in early 1989. The administrative offices are expected to be in operation in late 1988.

Konishiroku's investment in the project will total $120 million. Eighty percent of this amount will be committed in the United States.

The Konishiroku plant will represent the largest initial investment ever made by a Japanese company in North Carolina, according to Governor James G. Martin.

Initially, two-thirds of all raw materials to be used in production will be purchased from U.S. suppliers.

The plant will employ a work force of 250 to 300.

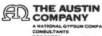

THE AUSTIN COMPANY
A NATIONAL GYPSUM COMPANY
CONSULTANTS
DESIGNERS
ENGINEERS
CONSTRUCTORS

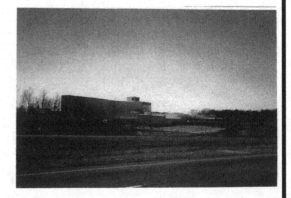

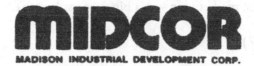

MADISON INDUSTRIAL DEVELOPMENT CORP.

April 10, 1987

Ronald F. Doyle
The Austin Company
3650 Mayfield Road
Cleveland, Ohio 44121

Dear Mr. Doyle:

Enclosed please find a gift from the City of Madison presented
at the Arvin Sango groundbreaking ceremony April 8, 1987.

On August 29, 1986, you first contacted me regarding this
project. The community is very happy that Arvin Sango Inc.
chose Madison as its headquarters. On behalf of the community,
I want to express our sincere gratitude to you and the Austin
Company for the professionalism and assistance in making this
all happen. The community is indebted to you and your firm. I
have appreciated the opportunity to work with you on this
project and offer you an open invitation to Madison to enjoy
with us the fruits of your labor.

Sincerely,

ROBERT M. EADS
President

jks

Enclosure

301 EAST MAIN STREET • MADISON, INDIANA 47250

AUSTIN MARKET PLAN (1986)

I was reassigned for the next few months to assist on an internal market definition plan with Bob Will and Harry Schlafmann. The market plan was a big success; I wasn't.

MY LAST STUDY (1987)

I worked on this favorable area study. But, by now, my light had dimmed . . . Were I a light bulb, I would be starting to flicker.

I was given the option by my management of three employment plans for the future: Leave now; leave in two weeks; or, leave in a month. I selected the middle option.

I received a warm going away party (luncheon) at a fine Japanese restaurant in Cleveland Heights, many handshakes, some good wishes . . . I left The Austin Company headquarters building August 14, 1987 as quietly as I had come in about 14 years before. I never returned, not even to visit.

PUBLISHED AUTHOR

FACILITIES LOCATION

R · E · V · I · E · W

A QUARTERLY ANALYSIS BY THE AUSTIN COMPANY OF A KEY FACILITY LOCATION TOPIC   SPRING 1987

WHERE WILL OUR CHILDREN WORK?

Ronald F. Doyle
Senior Location Consultant
Facilities Location Department

Introduction

During 1981 The Austin Company made an extensive study of state and regional variations and trends in average hourly earnings of manufacturing workers from 1962 through 1980. This study was subsequently published in the July/August 1982 issue of *Industrial Development* and was discussed at length in the November 1982 plenary session of the Industrial Development Research Council.

Among the more significant findings were

1. That average hourly earnings differences between Northern and Southern workers remained fairly consistent in "constant" dollars (adjusted for inflation) during the study period, and actually increased in current dollar terms.

2. That the average hourly production worker wage gap between Midwestern workers particularly and both New England and Western Sunbelt workers seems to be widening toward

The study concluded that the diffusion of manufacturing production out of the Northern States would continue but that the South would experience increasing competition from New England and the Western Sunbelt states for this production share.

With data now available for the first half of the 1980s and with the U.S. economy largely recovered from a recession and other economic shocks occurring since the study was made it appears to be an appropriate time to reassess the future outlook.

Employment Megatrends and The Manufacturing Sector (1980 - 1995)

Significant readjustments have occurred in the relationships between the manufacturing sector and the rest of the economy in terms of employment since 1980. Overall,

AVERAGE HOURLY EARNINGS IN MANUFACTURING VS RATE OF TOTAL EMPLOYMENT GROWTH (1980 - 1985)

UTILITY SPOTLIGHT

Published Since 1928

Vol. XXXVIII, No. 14   April 3, 1986

Inside
- Government Ban GE — p. 2
- Hydro Bills Viewed — p. 2
- Wrightsville Chief Out — p. 2
- Consumer Rate Qualified — p. 2
- Rate Settlement Reached — p. 3
- Gold Resources CEO — p. 3
- E&G Stocks Strong — p. 4

NUCLEAR COSTS SEEN SPURRING CORPORATE ELECTRICITY RATES

The cost of nuclear power continues to exert its still Ronald F. Doyle, author of a new study, and nuclear costs will be the catalyst behind future electricity rate increases for many of the "nation's largest corporations" — averaging somewhere in the neighborhood of 25% to 80% by 1990.

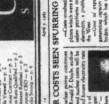

DOYLE

Doyle noted that electric power costs are likely to rise more rapidly than other traditional plant operating factors as the price of safer, cleaner and more abundant electric power is passed on to the consumer.

And still rising costs rears its ugly head in Doyle's study. He noted that anticipated legislation on the battle against air pollution, "especially in the midwest could result in substantially larger expenditures for pollution-control equipment at coal-fired generating facilities.

According to Doyle, who a senior location consultant for Austin, the projected increase will reflect the following:

— The expense of super public-utility commissions very favored into the study too. Doyle said the level and rate of increases will depend on some PUC's decisions to allow gradual rate increases over a period of years, while others will permit an immediate rate escalation. Then there

— Costs involved in unfinished nuclear plants which were mothballed because of either problems or lack of demand for electricity, a problem most prevalent in the West.

— Cost of expanding conventional generating capacity such as coal, lignite, hydro, which has occurred primarily in the Sun Belt states.

are those PUC's that will be motivated by what Doyle describes as "politically acceptable times" for rate hikes, which for example, would ultimately make utilities start purchasing for a highly lucrative contract such as the currently much sought after Saturn plant of General Motors Corp.

Doyle said on a regional basis, the costs showed that utilities in New England and California will continue to charge the highest rates and "Florida, Georgia and Alabama will have rates higher "than most other U.S. areas." "Costs will be moderate in the central U.S., but "considerably" rates are expected in the Pacific Northwest and Southern Plains.

Lower costs increases will be limited primarily in the region served by the Tennessee Valley Authority and the central Gulf Coast, Doyle added.

Some of the utilities surveyed in the Austin study include Alabama Power, Consumers Power, Duke Power Co., Gulf States Utilities, Iowa Electric Light & Power, Mississippi Power, Niagara Mohawk Power, Pacific Gas & Electric, Texas Utilities and Southern California Edison.

INDUSTRIAL DEVELOPMENT

JULY/AUGUST 1982

Past and Projected Labor Cost Trends in the U.S.

by Ronald F. Doyle

This study uses changes in wage rates within states and regions support some of our "conventional wisdom," but it also explodes a number of myths on wage rate changes in the Sunbelt and the Frostbelt.

ISSN 0019-9834

STOCK OFFER

THE AUSTIN COMPANY

STOCK SUBSCRIPTION AGREEMENT

The undersigned, an employee of The Austin Company (the "Company"), hereby subscribes for **400** shares of the Common stock of the Company ("Austin common stock") pursuant to all of the terms and provisions of the EMPLOYEE STOCK PURCHASE PLAN (the "Plan") of the Company, reference to which is hereby made as if all the terms and provisions thereof were fully set forth herein.

The undersigned agrees to pay the sum of $42.85 for each share covered by this Subscription Agreement, and full payment shall be made on or before April 28, 1985, with minimum installment payments to be made on said full payment in accordance with Section 2.01 of the Plan. Upon payment in full of this Subscription Agreement, the Company will deliver the total number of shares set forth herein registered in the name of the undersigned.

The undersigned's right to revoke and withdraw his deposit of funds hereunder and under the Plan as well as the automatic termination of this Subscription Agreement upon the undersigned's resignation, discharge, retirement or death shall be as set forth in ARTICLE III of the Plan. This Subscription Agreement is nonassignable.

Dated this ___7th___ day of May, 1990, at Cleveland Heights, Ohio.

_____
Employee's Signature

RONALD F. DOYLE
(Please print name)

ACCEPTED:

THE AUSTIN COMPANY

By: _____
A. A. Wilhelm, Vice President

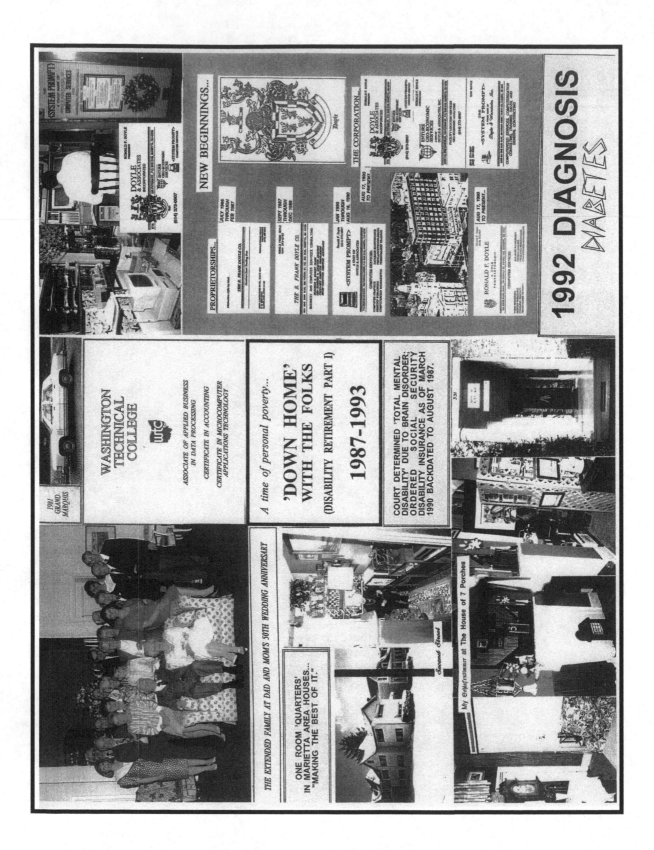

1992 DIAGNOSIS DIABETES

NEW BEGINNINGS...

PROPRIETORSHIPS...

THE CORPORATION...

WASHINGTON TECHNICAL COLLEGE

ASSOCIATE OF APPLIED BUSINESS IN DATA PROCESSING

CERTIFICATE IN ACCOUNTING

CERTIFICATE IN MICROCOMPUTER APPLICATIONS TECHNOLOGY

A time of personal poverty...

'DOWN HOME' WITH THE FOLKS
(DISABILITY RETIREMENT PART I)
1987-1993

COURT DETERMINED 'TOTAL MENTAL DISABILITY' DUE TO BRAIN DISORDER; ORDERED SOCIAL SECURITY DISABILITY INSURANCE AS OF MARCH 1990 BACKDATED TO AUGUST 1987.

THE EXTENDED FAMILY AT DAD AND MOM'S 50TH WEDDING ANNIVERSARY

ONE ROOM 'QUARTERS' IN MARIETTA AREA HOUSES... "MAKING THE BEST OF IT."

1981 GRAND MARQUIS

My Enhusiasm at The House of 7 Porches

CHAPTER FIVE
TOTAL DISABILITY

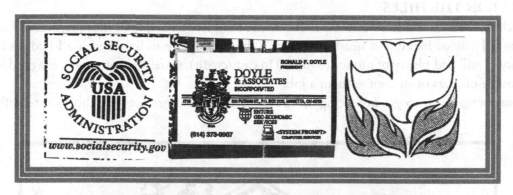

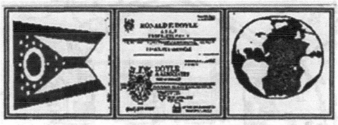

TOTAL DISABILITY: |
Down Home with the Folks
New Beginnings
A Renewal

(1987-1993): 10% OF MY LIFE BEFORE AGE 62

DOWN HOME WITH THE FOLKS

I settled in Marietta, Ohio (directly across the river from where I had spent my adolescent years and where my parents still lived) in September of 1987, and immediately began attending Washington Technical College (studying computers updating my technical skills), put together a small (tiny) business, and began a new period of my life: "down-home mid-life". At my request, the federal government thoroughly investigated my past and current circumstances, and I won a small settlement from court action. I worked some, rested some, and enjoyed much—for awhile anyhow. When I first came to Marietta, I lived in a small "college room" at a local bed and breakfast. Later, I had my own very modest three-room flat which I called 'The Hillside Hideaway' where I lived with my growing family of fish and my finch named Tweety Bird. My (business) workshop was in nearby downtown. I stayed now pretty much to myself, my family, and a small circle of school/business/club related friends. I was now intentionally discriminating in my associations; my exploring drives muted by realization of the limitations of age, disability advancement, and a more sober maturity. I was semi-retired due to these disabilities and had been made comfortable. But, I was reasonably happy at last for the time being.

BACK IN THE HILLS

Back in the hills, I adjusted to the Folks' home for a few days. Then, more recovered from the operation, I started looking in nearby Marietta, Ohio for a place to live. Because I had decided to 'lose face,' I still had plenty of money ($50,000 in cash/credit). Carefully conserved, it would last me for a couple of years or so even without a job.

A major goal was to get my racing mind slowed down and get over the shocks (mental) I had taken . . .

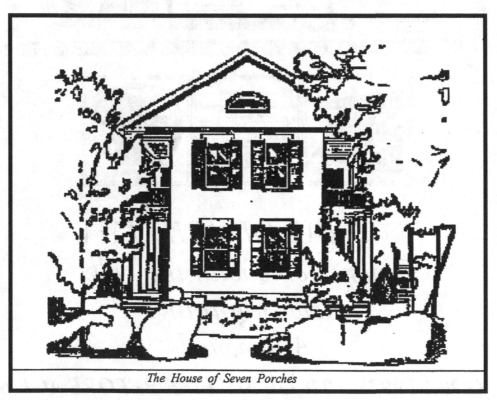

The House of Seven Porches

THE HOUSE OF SEVEN PORCHES

I succeeded in renting a room temporarily in a quaint historical house that had been converted into a bed and breakfast in Marietta, The House of Seven Porches, through the intercession of the local trade school housing assistance person. The place was well-suited for my needs at that time: it was not my father's house; it allowed an unadvertised entrance to living in Marietta (my emotional state being what it was I did not need the pressures of social scrutiny); it was adequate for my basic creature comforts; the owner, Jeane Kelso, lived there too and this gave me both company and a local reference as to my general character.

There, I had my 'college room' in the back upstairs. Although very small, it nevertheless sufficed. I decorated it with some of my things (the rest stored at my father's house) and adjusted to it. About the only 'negative' about the place was its gas stove heater. Eventually, I learned to use it also. It was a good place to live and the (low) negotiated month-to-month price was right.

WASHINGTON TECHNICAL COLLEGE ("Tinker Tech")

I, like many others, have discovered that if I am unable to work effectively at a career-level job (because of the mental acuity required for about 8 hours/day, about 5 days/week), I am yet able to attend school. School offers a variable workload (controlled by the student), variable attendance needs, and then only for about an hour at a time usually (requiring just a short attention span). It also offers long and more frequent breaks daily, and far more "vacation time" (breaks between quarters/semesters) than does nearly any kind of fulltime remunerative work.

Time spent at school with a little planning is seldom wasted . . . and prepares one for additional competitive opportunities once energy and other health/spiritual aspects improve sufficiently to reenter the workforce at whatever level prepared for.

I enrolled at WTC at the suggestion of the local government job service. A job for a completely "OK" person is difficult to find in Appalachia. I was already 'overqualified' in some respects, but lacked training at a trade.

Once enrolled, I used this time to do what my time on the road for Austin had prevented me from doing before—learn all I could about computers, software, and related topics. This knowledge gained at a pace I could absorb things, would bring me back into 'current times,' whether I ever went back into consulting or moved into some other field.

My association with this school I will always remember favorably because it suited my needs and pace at the time. (But, this school has now become Washington State Community College on another campus with a different atmosphere.)

MY SOLE PROPRIETORSHIP

In preparation for the possible loss of my career job in Cleveland, I had founded a tiny side venture known as 'The Coast-to-Coast Trading Post' as a sole proprietorship. In Cleveland, it was a mail-order company.

When I moved to Marietta, I restructured, changed its name, first, to do business consulting, and later to allow me to use my growing expertise at computers to do 'pilot projects' in programming, desktop publishing, and miscellaneous computer-related fields. Having the business set up allowed me to do some 'loss minimizing' work (new income against expenses) while attending school, recovering from previous strains, and exploring my new present and future. It also allowed me to do some more serious ancillary consulting in conjunction with active contacts sill in the facility location field. (I was able to do some minor work on two major plant location projects done mostly through another consultant.)

Eventually, I set up my headquarters in a local bank building and incorporated. Over the following years the physical plant (though small) and my useable corporate property grew into a comfortable, functional, corporate space.

'TOTAL MENTAL DISABILITY'

Beginning in 1988, I was advised by concerned medical advisors who had now come to notice me to seek SSDI as my condition was regarded by them as not permitting me to work. Working with a lawyer, I went methodically through the routine appeals process of Social Security. In late 1989, I had a hearing before an administrative law judge. In March 1990, I was awarded disability status dating back to August 1987 when I left the Austin Company. With the award money, I paid off some of my debts and put the rest into my business for if and when I recovered sufficiently to earn my living again. Minor commitments to studies at the technical college and "pilot projects" through my proprietorship continued as I kept busy at levels I thought I could and should.

A SHORT VACATION

In December 1990, I visited friends in North Carolina, a married couple I had known from Cleveland days. During the visit and on the way back, I visited 'The Lost Colony' in North Carolina and later Colonial Williamsburg in Virginia.

Outside of Norfolk one evening as darkness settled in I found myself asking directions. I pulled over into a parking lot to talk with a man parked there, ask him, smoke a cigarette, and stretch my legs . . .

It was just before the Gulf War. The young man about 25, had "Armed Forces" written all over him. We talked about the imminent situation (he wanted to). He was returning to Michigan to see his wife and small children . . . Sensing his uneasiness (angst), I sardonically tested his resolve, and he quickly responded that he would soon return and ship out with his unit to the Gulf.

I beheld his spirit. He simply wanted to know that Joe Citizen (who to him I apparently was) rapports him in what he and his fellows were about to do for us. He wanted 'permission' (Normal gentle people need this!)

To my mind, a mysterious message came in loud and clear. "Don't mess this up!"

I thought way back . . . to 1968.

I looked into his eyes which were staring wide openly at mine. With my eyes soft toward him yet steel blue, I said to him: "Kill them." (meaning the Iraqi enemy soldiers, if so ordered).

He reflected. Acknowledgement followed internally within him. He was now properly dispatched.

I did not know him personally; we had just met. The real reason I did that I later reflected was because I just wanted someone caught in the crunch of world history to be dispatched a little more gently, truthfully, and positively than I had been.

I wished him well. Very soon afterward we parted, each going our separate ways.

THE GULF WAR

I returned to Marietta. I put up a yellow ribbon next to a U.S. flag in my office. I decorated my computer with an American flag and a Sadam mimic: "The Mother of 386's," and listened to the news on radio and TV.

This seemed to pass as 'patriotism' to some onlookers. It wasn't. It was just courtesy and caring. Patriotism to me is the willingness to go forward to the battle oneself.

TWILIGHT TIMES: 1991-1993

I lived the next three years mostly withdrawn from society, sharing my time with my parents and family and some friends. I lived in Marietta, continuing to reside at The House of Seven Porches, and later in a small apartment. In my business, using some of the award money, I added to a modest physical plant more functional assets. I engaged in pilot projects and developed (hopefully) workable concepts for ultimately enlarging the business. Meanwhile, however, I grappled with variable dimness of mind and spirit accompanying my declined self-esteem that came from living in disguised 'failure'. Twilight began to envelope me as I wondered why I continued to live . . .

At this time, there were many good memories, and some sad ones, too. There was still my family and a few hard won old friends. There were also a couple of new friends, too. There was not as much money, but enough for the time being . . . though my credit was about exhausted and I was carrying a heavy debt/income ratio with interest payments straining me. But, overall, I was "comfortable". Life appeared *calm* to me, but I was having dread imaginings/premonitions about (my) imminent death. I decided that I really didn't care one way or the other if I died now. Trying to see a purpose for me beyond the next day's scheduled events, I could not . . . ANYTHNG was OK with me.

Suddenly, I was *really jolted* . . .

MY FATHER'S DEATH

I had joined the Folks Christmas morning for Mass at St Michael's where they usually attended church. My father and mother not wishing to travel far during the Christmas Holidays 1993 accepted my invitation to Christmas dinner at my place in Marietta. In the afternoon, they both arrived at my apartment. Mom had cooked most of the meal in her kitchen, together we finished cooking it at my place. I provided the accoutrements.

We had a pleasant afternoon together. A light snow was falling. A glance outside showed a pristinely beautiful white Christmas Day. As the Folks left I hugged them both only at that moment realizing how much I loved them, and how much they loved me. Then, they left. I cleaned up some. Then, I sat down. I was in an emotional pit I hoped I'd die soon. I seemed to have no further purpose.

Suddenly, the telephone rang. A woman's voice on the other end told me my parents had been involved in a one-car accident. Would I please come?

I arrived at the accident scene by the old Boaz bridge, about 10 minutes drive from their home. I darted between where emergency personnel were trying to remove my father from his vehicle to where my mother was resting with her injuries in a nearby house trailer.

I went with them to the hospital, following the ambulances. I stayed with my father, then my mother. Outside, weather conditions worsened. My father's condition was reportedly critical with no local doctor available to treat him. I agreed to let him be transported to Morgantown. And I took my mother, now discharged, to her home. My brothers now arrived. Vince and his wife Margie went immediately to Morgantown. Tim surveyed our situation and stayed with us.

Dad, died the next day. There was an evening funeral service at the funeral home a few days later. The day after that a Mass at St Michael's was said attended by many of his friends and relatives now filtering into town in the wintry weather to pay their last respects. My visions proliferated as I muddled through my role in my first *deep* sadness.

ANOTHER DAWN (The End of My Younger Life)

I'll remember Dad for having been my only reliable, consistent, dependable, loving, man-friend and father. The rest of the family and friends, although also caring, were less able to relate to me.

A realization finally sinks in from my father's repeated talks about his 'living on borrowed time'. We are all living on borrowed time. The 'loan' comes from God.

And as for the future I resolved to accept it a day at a time as it comes in the spirit of:

"Hard things I do right away. The impossible takes a little longer."

A VISITATION

In the immediate time span after my father's funeral I experienced an ultimate religious experience. This happened in such a way that it is impossible for my mind to even suggest that it didn't happen. The Holy Spirit came: Tersely I was chewed out for my failings—but surprisingly briefly. Just when I thought I'd die, instead, a feeling of serene peace descended upon me and up welled from inside me. God had chastised me. Then, He gave me peace! Apparently, I had failed to accomplish whatever mission in life had been mine. But, God loved me anyway and gave me evidence . . . I reawakened gradually over the ensuing years to know that for awhile yet mine would be a life worth living. And, no matter what my verdict at the entrance to the Afterlife will be, I now knew two things for certain: God is real. Christianity is true.

I wondered what this "New Day' would bring . . .

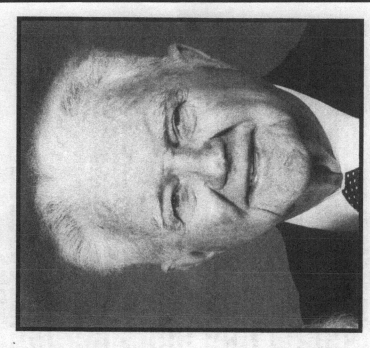

In Memorium

VINCENT LEO DOYLE

Born: January 26, 1909
Died: December 27, 1993

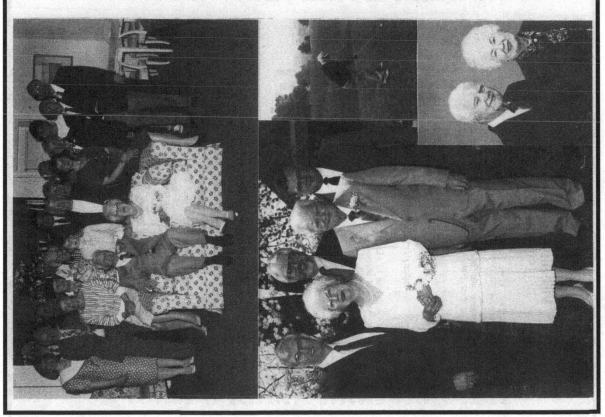

Eulogy
Vincent Leo Doyle
(1909-1993)

Written by his sons Tim, Vince, and Ron Doyle and delivered at Vinnie's funeral Mass on December 30, 1993.

Five years ago we gathered with friends and loved ones in a celebration of life with Vinnie and Irma at their 50th Anniversary.

Now we come together again today not to mourn his death, but to celebrate the beginning of the afterlife for Vinnie.

He touched many of us throughout his life, always there to lend a helping hand...

His early work with the dozens of kids he coached in Little League; the work and support he provided at Church; his active participation in projects with the boosters at Parkersburg Catholic High School, and most recently during his retirement, the pleasure and comraderie he shared with his many golfing partners at the Worthington Golf Club.

As a young man in Kearney, N.J. and one of the eldest of nine brothers and sisters remaining home after his mother passed away, he helped raise his younger brother Jim and sisters Dorothy and Mildred. He was also an avid athlete playing semi-pro baseball and soccer. He gave up a promising athletic career to dedicate his life to his wife and family. This would span his 47 year career with DuPont and his almost 20 years in retirement.

He was a master craftsman with practical solutions. "The difficult," he would say, "could be done right away...the impossible would take just a little longer."

His love of athletics fostered his competitive drive and feisty spirit. He had a zest for life and a compassion for people. He provided constant support and encouragement to his family and friends. He was the spiritual rock that provided family stability and yielded three fine "chips" in his sons.

We loved him and will miss him, but have many memories that we will treasure forever.

As he begins his journey to the afterlife, we bid him farewell.

"May the road rise up to meet you,
May the wind be always at your back,
May the sun shine warm upon your face,
and until we meet again,
May God hold you in the Hollow of His Hands."

P.S.   And may you be a long time in heaven before the devil knows you're gone!

THE HOMILY AT THE FUNERAL MASS

Written and delivered by Fr. Anthony Conlon, St. Michael's Parish, Vienna, WV.

"You would have suffered eternal death had He not been born in time. Never would you have been freed of sinful flesh. You would have suffered everlasting unhappiness had it not been for this mercy. You never would have returned to life had He not shared your death. You would have been lost had He not hastened to your aid. You would have perished had He not come." So wrote St. Augustine of Hippo many centuries ago.

Once a woman said to me as she was undergoing great sorrow and trials, "Wouldn't it be awful if God had not come into the world--life would have no meaning." Vincent Doyle's earthly life came to an end during the Christmas season, when we celebrate the entry of God into the world in human flesh and blood. Vincent took the truths of his faith and wove them into his daily life and work. It was this that went to make the fabric of his life. If Vincent wasn't at Mass on Sunday with a big handshake as he came through the door, he was either sick or on the road.

Vincent has entered into eternal life and now we look to ourselves for "we must be talking to ourselves." The Son of Man was glorified in His death and resurrection. The Gospel reading puts it: "Unless the grain of wheat falls to the earth and dies, it remains just a grain of wheat (John). Strange how, from death comes life. One of these Christian paradoxes.

When preparing the children for First Communion I bring them up around the altar and put some altar bread in the sacred vessels. Then, I ask, "How do you get bread?" We go back to the beginning where the earth is plowed and prepared. Then the seed is dropped into the earth and covered. Then I ask what happens to the seed. And invariably they will say "it grows". But, I continue to ask what happens to the seed. Eventually they come to see that it dies. It has to die to grow and produce more wheat.

So it is with you and I. We die many times. We die to the comfort and security of life in our mothers' wombs in order to be born into the world. That is quite a traumatic experience, only in the end to find ourselves surrounded by loving people. We die to the comfort and security of youth to move out into the world and make our way through it. We die to the comfort and security and affections our children return to us to enjoy a different form of life. And in the end, it is in dying that we are born to eternal life.

The same thing is said of the Church. The Church is dying it is said. Of course, the Church is dying. The Church is always dying. But, the Church is always rising, too. In all of this another great Christian paradox is brought home to us when Christ says: "The one who loves his life loses it, while the one who hates his life in this world preserves it to life eternal."

In all of this I am reminded of the words of Patrick H. Pierce in his poem, *The Fool:*

"...I have squandered the splendid years which the Lord God gave to my youth in attempting impossible things.
Was it folly or grace?
Not men shall judge me but God.
I have squandered the splendid years.
Lord, if I had the years I would squander them over again.
Aye!   Fling them from me.
For this I have heard in my heart
That a man shall scatter, not hoard,
Shall do the deed of today, nor take thought of tomorrow's teen,
Shall not bargain or huckster with God."

We follow Vincent with our prayers that he will now enjoy the perfect happiness of heaven, and that one day we will merit to join him.

APPENDIX

WASHINGTON TECHNICAL COLLEGE

1987-1991

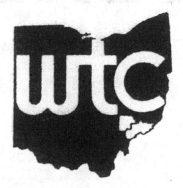

ASSOCIATE of APPLIED BUSINESS DEGREE
Data Processing Technology
Conferred 12/08/1989

CERTIFICATE
Accounting
Conferred 6/08/1990

CERTIFICATE
Microcomputer Applications Technology
Conferred 6/14/1991

Washington State COMMUNITY COLLEGE

OFFICE OF THE REGISTRAR
710 Colegate Drive
Marietta, Ohio 45750

Michael D. Whitmable, Registrar

ACADEMIC RECORD OF:	Doyle, Ronald F
ADDRESS	331 Fifth Street, Marietta OH 45750
STUDENT NUMBER	235-70-8053
DATE OF BIRTH:	May 02
DATE PRINTED:	February 27, 2003
ACADEMIC LEVEL:	Undergraduate

Issued To Student

COURSE NUMBER	TITLE	CREDIT HOURS	GRADE	QUALITY POINTS
FALL '87 (09/21/1987 to 12/12/1987)				
00600 151 01	DESIGN DRAFT I	5.00	B	9.00
00160 132 01	INTRO DP/BASIC	4.00	A	16.00
00600 241 01	CAD I	4.00	A	16.00
ENG 416	COMP (540 111)	5.00	X	0.00
MATH 459	ALGEBRA/TRIG (450 109)	5.00	X	0.00
ECON 501	ECONOMICS (570 211)	3.00	X	0.00
ACCT 501	ACCOUNTING I (100 151)	4.00	X	0.00
ACCT 502	ACCOUNTING II (100 152)	4.00	X	0.00
SOC 507	SOCIOLOGY (680 211)	3.00	X	0.00
BUS 621	BUSINESS LAW (120 166)	4.00	X	0.00
ENG 418	COMP (540 112)	0.00	X	0.00
ENG 417	COMP (540 112)	4.00	X	0.00
	OHIO STATE UNIVERSITY			
ATT 11.00	ERN 41.00 QUAL PTS 41.00		GPA	3.727
CUM 11.00	ERN 41.00 QUAL PTS 41.00		GPA	3.727
WINTER '88 (01/04/1988 to 03/19/1988)				
00160 142 01	ADVANCED BASIC	4.00	A	16.00
00160 241 01	INTRO TO COBOL	4.00	B	12.00
00120 156 70	BUSINESS MGT II	3.00	A	12.00
00600 242 01	CAD II	4.00	A	16.00
	DEAN'S LIST			
ATT 15.00	ERN 15.00 QUAL PTS 56.00		GPA	3.733
CUM 26.00	ERN 56.00 QUAL PTS 97.00		GPA	3.731
SPRING '88 (03/28/1988 to 06/10/1988)				
00160 242 01	ADVANCED COBOL	4.00	C	8.00
00160 251 70	PC SYSTEM TECHNIQ	4.00	B	12.00
00160 252 02	INTRO TO LOTUS 1-2-3	4.00	A	16.00
ATT 12.00	ERN 12.00 QUAL PTS 36.00		GPA	3.000
CUM 38.00	ERN 68.00 QUAL PTS 133.00		GPA	3.500

Continued on next Column/Page

COURSE NUMBER	TITLE	CREDIT HOURS	GRADE	QUALITY POINTS
SUMMER I '88 (06/20/1988 to 08/26/1988)				
00120 157 70	SMALL BUS ENTREP	4.00	A	16.00
00120 155 01	BUSINESS MGT I	3.00	B	9.00
00120 145 70	BUSINESS TYPING	5.00	C	6.00
00540 115 70	TECH WRITING	4.00	A	16.00
00650 165 01	BUSINESS MATH	5.00	X	0.00
ATT 14.00	ERN 19.00 QUAL PTS 47.00		GPA	3.357
CUM 52.00	ERN 87.00 QUAL PTS 180.00		GPA	3.462
FALL '88 (09/19/1988 to 12/09/1988)				
00650 122 70	DATA MATH	4.00	A	16.00
00160 151 01	INTRO RPG II	4.00	B	12.00
00160 252 01	ADV PROG & LANG	4.00	B	12.00
ATT 12.00	ERN 12.00 QUAL PTS 40.00		GPA	3.333
CUM 64.00	ERN 99.00 QUAL PTS 220.00		GPA	3.438
WINTER '89 (01/03/1989 to 03/17/1989)				
00200 247 70	ADV WORD PROC	0.00	W	0.00
00160 152 01	ADVANCED RPG II	4.00	C	8.00
00120 166 01	BUSINESS LAW I	0.00	W	0.00
00540 117 70	BUS WRITING	4.00	A	16.00
00100 281 95	MICROCOMP ACCT	0.00	F	0.00
ATT 12.00	ERN 8.00 QUAL PTS 24.00		GPA	2.000
CUM 72.00	ERN 107.00 QUAL PTS 244.00		GPA	3.389
SPRING '89 (03/27/1989 to 06/09/1989)				
00160 245 01	COMP OPER & UTIL	4.00	A	16.00
00160 200 64	INTR WORDPERFECT 5.0	1.00	S	0.00
00160 200 66	EXCEL	1.00	S	0.00
00160 200 67	DBASE III PLUS	1.00	S	0.00
00160 233 01	BUS SYSTEM DSGN	4.00	L	16.00
00550 151	SPEECH	4.00	L	

Washington State
COMMUNITY COLLEGE

OFFICE OF THE REGISTRAR
710 Colegate Drive
Marietta, Ohio 45750

Michael D. Whitnable, Registrar

DATE PRINTED: February 27, 2003
ACADEMIC LEVEL: Undergraduate

ACADEMIC RECORD OF: Doyle, Ronald F

ADDRESS: 331 Fifth Street
Marietta OH 45750

STUDENT NUMBER: 235-70-8053

DATE OF BIRTH: May 02

Issued to Student

COURSE NUMBER	TITLE	CREDIT HOURS	GRADE	QUALITY POINTS
ATT 8.00	ERN 15.00 QUAL PTS 32.00		GPA	4.000
CUM 80.00	ERN 122.00 QUAL PTS 276.00		GPA	3.450
SUMMER I '89 (06/19/1989 to 08/25/1989)				
00100 153 85	PRIN ACCT III	4.00	B	12.00
00100 281 85	MICROCOMP ACCT	4.00	B	12.00
00100 282 85	SPREADSHEET ACCT	3.00	C	6.00
ATT 11.00	ERN 11.00 QUAL PTS 30.00		GPA	2.727
CUM 91.00	ERN 133.00 QUAL PTS 306.00		GPA	3.363
FALL '89 (09/18/1989 to 12/08/1989)				
00200 247 02	WORDPERFECT 5.0	4.00	C	8.00
ATT 4.00	ERN 4.00 QUAL PTS 8.00		GPA	2.000
CUM 95.00	ERN 137.00 QUAL PTS 314.00		GPA	3.305

Degree Received: Assoc Applied Bus
Date Conferred: 12/08/1989
Majors..........: Data Processing Tech

COURSE NUMBER	TITLE	CREDIT HOURS	GRADE	QUALITY POINTS
WINTER '90 (01/02/1990 to 03/16/1990)				
00110 241 20	MICROCOMPUTER DIAG	3.00	A	12.00
00110 251 20	LOCAL AREA NETWORKING	4.00	A	16.00
ATT 7.00	ERN 7.00 QUAL PTS 28.00		GPA	4.000
CUM 102.00	ERN 144.00 QUAL PTS 542.00		GPA	3.553
SPRING '90 (03/26/1990 to 06/08/1990)				
00110 271 20	NEW MICROCOMPUTER APPL	0.00	W	0.00
00120 167 70	BUSINESS LAW I1	4.00	B	12.00
ATT 4.00	ERN 4.00 QUAL PTS 12.00		GPA	3.000
CUM 106.00	ERN 148.00 QUAL PTS 354.00		GPA	3.340

Continued on next Column/Page

Degree Received: Certificate
Date Conferred.: 06/08/1990
Majors..........: Accounting Cert

COURSE NUMBER	TITLE	CREDIT HOURS	GRADE	QUALITY POINTS
FALL '90 (05/17/1990 to 12/07/1990)				
00150 200 63	MS-DOS II & WINDOWS	0.00	W	0.00
00110 261 85	WORD PROC & PUBLISHING	4.00	A	15.00
00500 226 70	MGT & SUPERVSN	4.00	A	16.00
00100 221 20	COST ACCT I	0.00	W	0.00
00110 210 20	DATABASE MANAGEMENT	0.00	W	0.00
	Mbr Phi Theta Kappa			
	Internat'l Honor Soci			
	(3.5 GPA required)			
ATT 8.00	ERN 8.00 QUAL PTS 32.00		GPA	4.000
CUM 114.00	ERN 156.00 QUAL PTS 386.00		GPA	3.536
WINTER '91 (01/07/1991 to 03/22/1991)				
00160 200 63	MS-DOS II & WINDOWS	1.00	A	4.00
00110 210 85	DATABASE MANAGEMENT	4.00	B	12.00
ATT 5.00	ERN 5.00 QUAL PTS 16.00		GPA	3.200
CUM 119.00	ERN 161.00 QUAL PTS 402.00		GPA	3.378
SPRING '91 (04/01/1991 to 06/14/1991)				
	NEW MAJOR: MICROCOMPU			
	APPLICATIONS			
00110 122 32	COMPUTER PROG II	0.00	R	0.00
ATT 0.00	ERN 0.00 QUAL PTS 0.00		GPA	0.000
CUM 119.00	ERN 161.00 QUAL PTS 402.00		GPA	3.378

Continued on next Column/Page

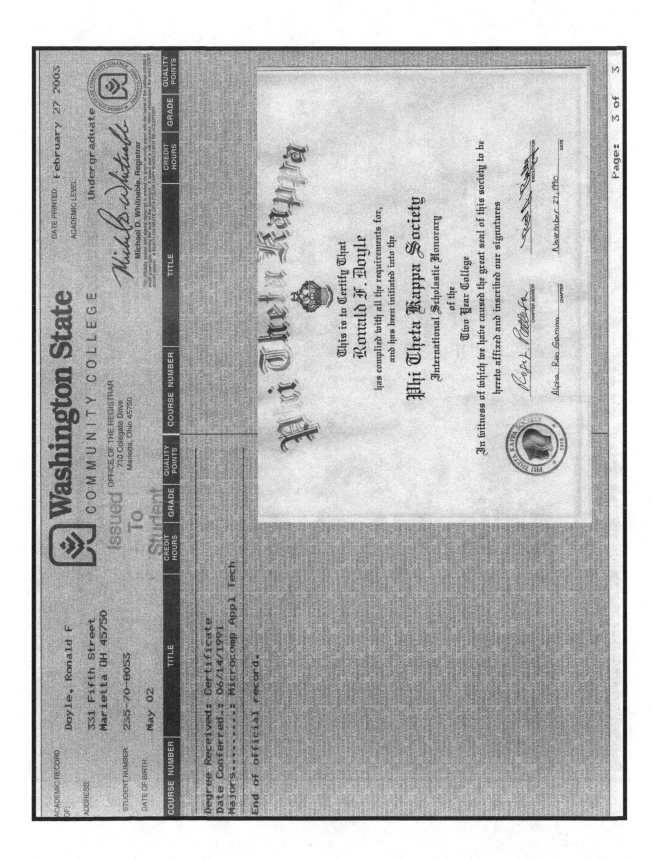

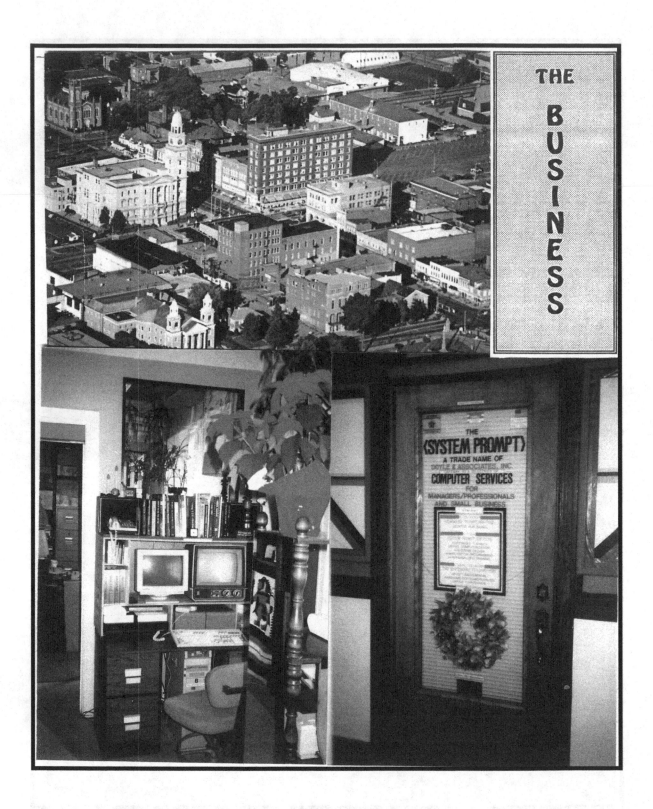

**THE HISTORY OF THE FREELANCE ENTREPRENEURIAL ACTIVITIES
OF RONALD FRANK DOYLE
Late 1986/Early 1987
THE R. FRANK DOYLE COMPANY**
The Coast-to-Coast Trading Post

Early Losses

The business was born The R. Frank Doyle Company (trade named The Coast-to-Coast Trading Post) in Euclid, Ohio in July of 1986. I used my middle name in an attempt to hide my "moonlighting" from my employer. But, I soon let them in on my venture. It started out in my apartment as a mail order company selling specialty gift and miscellaneous items out of catalogs. Friends at work and my family provided my first orders. I had no employees. The business was a flop losing much money in the first months. I closed it early in 1987.

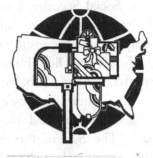

Logo

**Late 1987/1988-1989
THE R. FRANK DOYLE COMPANY
BUSINESS AND COMPUTERIZATION CONSULTING**

Small Profits

After being laid off at The Austin Company (which had been my fulltime employer), I returned to the Mid-Ohio Valley (my boyhood home). I quickly concentrated my efforts in two directions: I enrolled in Washington Technical College/Washington State Community College (WTC/WSCC) to learn as much about computers as I could as quickly as I could; and, I restructured my sole proprietorship to do "business and computerization consulting".

I located an office in the Dime Bank Building in Marietta. My former boss at Austin, Bob Will, then retired and working out of his North Carolina home, and Louis DeSappio of Executive Maintenance locally were my two main customers. I assisted Bob Will on two plant location studies for German manufacturers locating in the U.S.. The work for Bob met with marginal acceptance. I offered Louis DeSappio some of my opinions on his corporate policies and on office computerization. I was not very helpful as a business or computerization consultant, however. Later, I did some Lotus programming for Karmen's Grocery and that project, though small, went well. I also tried to do a job for Kevin Brown (Mullen Motors) but could not because I lacked enough computer knowledge.

Late in 1989 I withdrew from most business endeavors because my dementia interfered with my performance and I felt I needed the time at the tech school to learn more about computers.

**1990
THE
<SYSTEM PROMPT>
A UNIT OF
DOYLE & ASSOCIATES, INC.
COMPUTERIZATION CONSULTING**

More Training/Blue Sky!

This year saw me involved in receiving technical training at WTC/WSCC and only sporadically involved with the business. A court also officially declared me "totally mentally disabled" in March. Capital for my venture arrived in the form of an Award from Social Security. I set up the business for the long haul in facility location and computerization consulting by incorporating (with lawyer Dick Thomas' and CPA Jo Smith's help) as a Subchapter S corporation by the name of Doyle and Associates, Inc.. I trade named the computerization part "The System Prompt" and renamed my sole proprietorship "Ronald F. Doyle A.S.P." to be the asset holder. I also bought a state-of-the-art full 386 computer and peripheral equipment.

1991-1993

New Offices/Significant Losses

Accomplishments of the corporation were very minor. There were no facility location clients. Computerization work I limited to "pilot projects" in order to see what I could and could not do successfully.

Early in 1991, I renovated the corporate offices on the Seventh Floor of the Dime Bank. I finished my training at WTC/WSCC in that summer. In the fall, I began an office computerization job (a four figure project) for Dr. William Beatty in Columbus. And toward year's end, I moved my corporate headquarters down to renovated offices on the Sixth Floor of the Dime Bank.

The early part of 1992 saw me finish up the work for Beatty. The job was a "success". (I got paid.) I spent the rest of '92 and '93 doing small jobs successfully for various clients, and others and in thoroughly learning how to use my equipment. In early 1993, Harold Robbins of Kidstuff approached me to help him with a major (five figure) project: computerize his toy store. I tried to do this, accomplished some assistance with the help of Paul Bowles and another computer consultant who agreed to subcontract under me, but ultimately I could not do the work well enough. Robbins happily paid for what I had done but withdrew in favor of another provider.

Late in '93, I ceased searching for new major business . . .

1994 On

Ronald F. Doyle
A SOLE PROPRIETORSHIP
Dormancy

In December '93 and then again in August '94 I decided to withdraw from active business pursuits because my talents had precipitously decreased due to the shock of my father's passing and the return of bouts with mental illness and because my losses had become significant. I put my corporation "to sleep".

As a dormant business, I kept my offices and legal viability, but rented out office space to Bill Morris and later also Jack Ottenheimer (Yellow Cab). I continued to serve Bill Morris' small needs and did little jobs for Pauline Hines (NAMI/WC). At the end of 1999, I inactivated my corporation and devoted my sole proprietorship completely to subletting furnished office space at the WesBanco Building (formerly the Dime Bank Building) to Bill Morris and Jack Ottenheimer.

Shortly afterwards I fixed up office space for myself there to work on readings and written materials for the Ohio Community Support Planning Council. As Bill Morris became more enfeebled he prevailed upon me through my sole proprietorship to be his companion/caregiver until the end of his life in 2002. During this time I vacated the offices when the rent became too high. After Bill Morris died I ceased to do business at all and closed out the business checking account (2002).

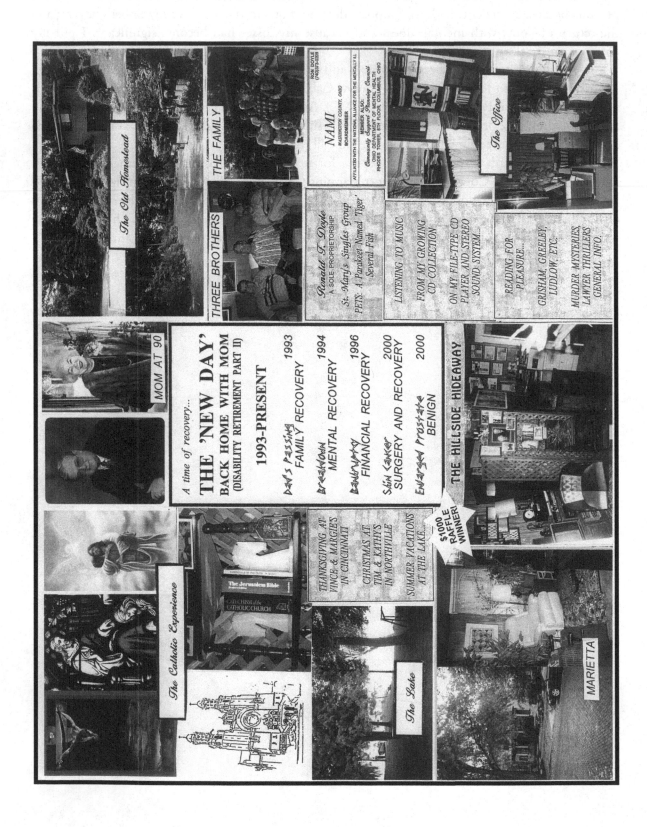

The Old Homestead

THE FAMILY

THREE BROTHERS

Ronald F. Doyle
A SOLE PROPRIETORSHIP
St. Mary's Singles Group
PETS: A Parakeet Named 'Tiger'
Several Fish

LISTENING TO MUSIC

FROM MY GROWING
CD COLLECTION

ON MY FILE-TYPE CD
PLAYER AND STEREO
SOUND SYSTEM...

RON DOYLE
(740)373-0209

NAMI
WASHINGTON COUNTY, OHIO
BOARDMEMBER

AFFILIATED WITH THE NATIONAL ALLIANCE FOR THE MENTALLY ILL

MEMBER, ALSO:
Community Support Planning Council
OHIO DEPARTMENT OF MENTAL HEALTH
RHODES TOWER, 8TH FLOOR, COLUMBUS, OHIO

The Office

READING FOR
PLEASURE...

GRISHAM, GREELEY,
LUDLOW, ETC.

MURDER MYSTERIES,
LAWYER THRILLERS,
GENERAL INFO.

MOM AT 90

A time of recovery...

THE 'NEW DAY'
BACK HOME WITH MOM
(DISABILITY RETIREMENT PART II)

1993-PRESENT

Dad's Passing   FAMILY RECOVERY   1993

Breakdown   MENTAL RECOVERY   1994

Bankruptcy   FINANCIAL RECOVERY   1996

Skin Cancer   SURGERY AND RECOVERY   2000

Enlarged Prostate   BENIGN   2000

THE HILLSIDE HIDEAWAY

$1000
RAFFLE
WINNER!

The Catholic Experience

The Jerusalem Bible

CATECHISM of the
CATHOLIC CHURCH

THANKSGIVING AT
VINCE & MARGIE'S
IN CINCINNATI

CHRISTMAS AT
TIM & KATHY'S
IN NORTHVILLE

SUMMER VACATIONS
AT THE LAKE...

The Lake

MARIETTA

CHAPTER SIX
THE NEWDAY

Christian Living
Mom's Last Hoorah
My Transition into 'Old Age'

(1994-2008): 23% OF MY LIFE BEFORE AGE 62

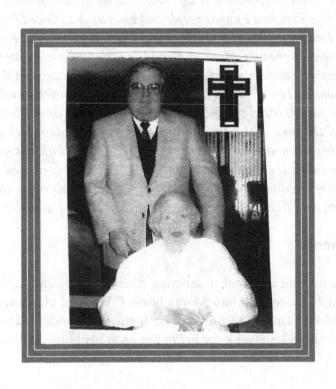

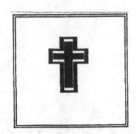

THE 'NEW DAY': CHRISTIAN LIVING &
'TRADING PLACES' WITH MY MOTHER

At my father's passing I was given to know (beyond doubt) that God is and had been with me throughout my younger years witnessing my life and generally protecting me. Life now changed as I was drawn closer to God. Gradually, I separated myself from vices that had occupied much time in my younger years. I foreswore frequent sex fantasies and even occasional drinking. Otherwise I also grew in the overall practice of the Catholic Faith. I benefited from God's graces and also enjoyed a life of easier living. But, my list of past flaws was long . . . Because I had been a bad manager of money, I lived in near poverty. Yet I wanted for nothing. I simply had no money in the bank. Schizophrenia and diabetes continued to affect my life. Yet these problems were largely controlled by medications and other health practices. On the other hand these illnesses did keep me both busy yet unfit to work. In the community I had no social status except maybe that of an "older unemployable mentally disabled unattached bachelor" and I was largely ignored by most people and completely excluded from "society".

At the beginning, I stayed mostly with my mother at The Old Homestead in Vienna so as to be able to care for her overall needs as she was elderly and could do little for herself. Later, becoming efficient at this, I began to live routinely mornings and nights at my mother's house, the Old Homestead, and late mornings and afternoons at The Hillside Hideaway, my place in Marietta and my legal residence.

These years simply passed. Mostly they were pleasant years. Aside from Mom and my brothers and their families, I passed the time with friends Bill Morris, Helen Jordan, Jack and Jan Ottenheimer, Pauline Hines and others. I mostly ceased "the Business" (1994) and all but abandoned my office at the Dime Bank (later called the WesBanco Building), subletting it furnished until I surrendered it entirely in 2001. Most of the time I spent divided taking care of Mom's needs, concentrating on taking care of my health needs, and filling the rest of the time as usefully as I was able to. I lived quietly.

Living Arrangements

With my father gone and my mother suffering from a stroke condition, my family prevailed upon me to immediately move back into Mom's house ("The Old Homestead") to look after her needs. (This allowed Mom to stay in Vienna with her house and friends for a little longer. She doesn't drive and it would have been impossible for her to live on at her house without me.).[1]

---

[1]   NOTE: 'God' referred to in this text is not a living, walking, talking Jesus but rather a 'Presence,' a light in my head, the Holy Spirit. Communication to me was by thought sequencing and the juxtaposing of feelings, not by words

So, at the age of 47, I moved into Mom's house, my boyhood home, and took over my brother's room! Since this was only supposed to be temporary I decided to keep my apartment ("The Hillside Hideaway") however.

Mom and I adjusted quickly to living together and to my going to my apartment every daytime. This practice gave each of us just enough personal space to keep at peace with each other and for me not to get bored.

Business Dormancy

Earning a living "outside the home" quickly dissipated as a goal as monetary pursuits just became unimportant (when compared to death in the family, etc.). I made a heroic stab at trying to keep the business going in 1994, but, after seeing the size of my losses, experiencing the mental strain, and concluding that I simply was not able to put enough quality time into the business because of my condition I decided to "cease". To be sure, I kept my legal viability as a Subchapter S corporation and kept my offices in the Dime Bank (Wesbanco Building), but I ceased to court new business and almost immediately I had no customers except Bill Morris and Jack Ottenheimer to whom I sublet office space and rented out equipment and for whom I did very small sporadic jobs.

After a severe psychotic break and hospitalization in August '94 (possibly a reaction to my father's death, irrational guilt feelings and work stress) I rested a bit then began to take an interest in part-time employment. But, jobs a consumer could do were scarce. I only really connected once, at Hardees working part-time as a salad preparer. There, finally in a job specifically designed for someone with a brain disorder, the stress of the physical grind 6 hours/day, 3 days/week quickly produced paranoia for some reason however and within a month I quit rather than go the route back to psychotic break which I am all too familiar with. I was out the door. A couple of days later I also noticed my arm hurting. What had happened was a rotator cuff injury possibly due to weakened muscles, a side effect of some of the anti-psychotic medication I took over the years. It was becoming apparent to me that almost all employment was out of the question—my disability was indeed total!

I got used to being satisfied with being totally "disability retired". I began to tell everyone that I was "retired" and I was generally accepted as such.

Personal Finances

I had virtually no money to my name. In 1994 I was also $25,000 in debt. In a legal maneuver (bankruptcy), I managed to get out from under this debt in the late 90's. But, even freed from heavy interest and principal payments, there was just enough income to pay bills.

Yet this income was sufficient. And, after all, I did little to earn it (for the most part). There were two parts to it: social security disability payments, and the pharmaceutical company's payments for my medicine. Mom supplied a car. Sporadically I also had a tiny income from subletting the offices or doing odd jobs through my "business". After 55, I also had pension money coming in. I figure, were I working and also having to pay taxes (As a disabled person I was largely tax exempt.) I would have to have gross wages of between $15,000-$20,000 per year plus have a good benefits package to have the same lifestyle as I was able to have during this period of my life.

Maintaining Single Status

In First Corinthians, Saint Paul says that if a man is sealed by the Holy Spirit while single he should stay single. But, it is no sin if he does marry. Nevertheless, as the years passed no eligible females entered my life, nor was I motivated to pursue marriage or even dating. It became apparent that I would continue to live single. Among other things, this meant that most activities I engaged in would be engaged in without a partner. As it worked out most activities I engaged in I engaged in alone.

Filling the Time

Filling the time usefully and enjoyably became the focus of my new life after dealing with my priorities.

My first priority, of course, was taking care of Mom, who as she became more elderly became also more enfeebled. Mostly I did the shopping and driving for her—shopping for all manner of items but especially food from the grocery stores and drugs from the drugstores, and driving her to the doctor's and the dentist's, etc..Twice each year (in the 1990's) I drove her (and myself) to Cincinnati or Detroit to visit my brothers. I also helped her with her shoes and stockings mornings and nights, set her hair occasionally, and performed numerous small unskilled tasks around her house. In exchange, because she was still able, she did her own cooking, kept track of the many medications for me and herself, and did our wash with help from me. We shared much time together because we wanted to and kept each other in company. We also watched each other's health.

I renewed my Catholic Faith—but not as a fanatic. I did, however, gradually get into the regiment of regular Mass and the Sacraments and, later, daily prayer and/or Scripture reading. I attended several religious functions and participated in many religious activities too through the Catholic Singles Group at St. Mary's. As money began to stretch further and when I occasionally had more money, I step-by-step increased my support of the Church and of other charities. I also solicited for charity in my neighborhood sporadically.

My main volunteer time involvement, however, was with the National Alliance for the Mentally Ill (NAMI) through Pauline Hines, where, for several years, I was a "board member" of NAMI/Washington county. The board meetings about every other month consisted of a conversational get-together to discuss mental health issues and news. An occasional support group meeting offered to the community-at-large was most often unattended. Through NAMI/WC I became in contact with NAMI/Ohio as well. Through NAMI/Ohio I became involved with the Ohio Community Support Planning Council in 2000 until the end of 2002. It mostly consisted of attending 5.5 hours of meeting time (divided by a one hour lunch break) once every 2 months to review and comment on mental health issues before the Ohio Department of Mental Health. The meetings were held in Columbus. I was "consumer" delegate (from SE Ohio). My contribution there was negligible, not really being able to keep up intellectually with many of the "normal" delegates.

I continued and expanded my friendships particularly with Helen Jordan and Bill Morris, two people many years my senior. I visited with them often and enjoyed many conversations on their lives and activities and my life and activities until their respective deaths.

While all of the above activities were done for my mental health and well-being, giving me a routine of light duty to follow which allowed me to progressively gain strength, specific tasks had to be accomplished regarding my medications and other direct health practices. Besides taking the medications on schedule (Mom helped much with this), I had to keep track of when the medications ran out, often fill out and submit new patient assistance forms, finger prick twice a day to take my sugar readings, constantly watch my diet, exercise regularly, make doctors' visits (GP, urologist, skin doctor, eye doctor, etc.), see the dentist, and see the psychiatrist (him also because the State of Ohio wanted me to after the break of '94).

The activities just mentioned did not occupy all of my time, however. The rest of my time, rather than let it hang on me, I filled with many solitary activities. Among other things these were principally:

Listening to music: I grew my CD collection carefully selecting what really appealed to me. Routinely I listened to my favorite selections mostly in the afternoons and often shared them with Mom and other guests at my apartment.

Watching TV: At The Hideaway I tuned in to CNN to keep abreast of the times. I also often watched TV at night with Mom.

Reading: I read and reread the Bible again and again, learning something new or comforting with each rereading. I also took to reading mystery novels, particularly the works of John Grisham. I could not read much at a time but I read a chapter or so a day, eventually reading many full books.

Writing/desktop publishing: I really got into writing this journal and publishing on the computer what I could. It occupied many hours figuring out the best ways to do things and was a joy to recount my many memories and experiences in print. Other than this book, there were occasional letters for Mom and myself, small jobs for Bill, and at one point a newsletter for Pauline Hines. Throughout I used WordPerfect 5.0 because I still remembered how to use the program from the training at WTC. I did manual cut and paste for pictures however. The newer programs were too complicated for my mind and "if it ain't broke, don't fix it."

Shopping: My income was high enough that I could spend a small amount each month on clothes or other things that I wanted but did not desperately need. However, I could not really waste a penny. I learned to thoroughly enjoy comparison shopping for bargains or inexpensive items. Wal-Mart became my favorite store. (But, for quality I occasionally found myself shopping at more expensive stores too.)

Fixing up the properties I rented: I had no money for large scale activities in this regard. But, I did enjoy fixing up The Hideaway and my WesBanco offices, buying inexpensive but attractive furnishings and doing the interior decorating.

Seasonal activities: May through September brought lawn and garden work at The Old Homestead. While there was more work requiring more physical and mental skills and abilities than I had to do here, I made my contribution. Ultimately I stopped all outside work because of my susceptibility to poison ivy and the reluctance of doctors to give me the shots to take it away because of my diabetes I think. December was filled with Christmas shopping and decorating my apartment. February brought taxes and the annual updating of my books for Jo Smith to do the taxes.

Contemplating: I contemplated the wonders of God and my life while eating out frequently by myself at area restaurants, or while drinking diet soda at home in the Florida room. Smoking time

(11/2 packs a day) was also contemplation time. Life slowed down to a pace where I could almost handle anything . . . When my sugar was up or when I felt groggy from the schizophrenia medicine I often snoozed on my La-Z-Boy in my apartment.

Surfing the Internet: After Mom got her computer I spent time learning how to surf. I never developed much interest however and used the Web mostly just for occasional information searches. Using the web impressed me as complicated.

Working for pay: Always on my mind, genuine opportunities that I could do in my condition simply did not exist. This door was mostly closed to me during the years with Mom. My business (which mostly consisted of subletting furnished office space) continued, however. It produced a tiny income periodically. Basically I could do most anything that didn't require speed with accuracy (limitations imposed by dementia and grogginess), didn't require heavy lifting, or constant movement (the need for frequent breaks). Quality was also a problem unless I could redo my work until I got it right. I could not do yard work because of poison ivy. I also needed to have a bathroom readily accessible because of my diabetes. In short, I as a worker would have been "more trouble than I was worth" to an employer—and employers knew it.

Caring for pets and plants: Tiger, the parakeet, seemed to thrive under Mom's and my care. Otherwise, I cared for fish in my aquariums first at Mom's house then later at the apartment. Usually, I had goldfish. I also bought and maintained many plants for The Hideaway.

THE 'NEW DAY'S SUNSET

As time continued to pass, I lived quietly content in my "no status" retired station, sharing in Mom's 'good situation' because she needed to have someone to live with her (and the family elected me), just caring for Mom and enjoying life one day at a time. I'd accept life as it came.

While I didn't get out of life what I had planned, I was happy and thankful for what I did get. In short, God had given me a 'nice long rest'—on "Easy Street," spending my time for the most part only with those people who loved and cared about me and about whom I loved and cared.

Then, in August 2003, the endings to this relatively easy life began as my mother's health slipped seriously. "Normal life" with its bigger challenges, worries and pain was about to return . . .

MOM'S LAST HOORAH
AND THE TRANSITION

This chapter summarizes my mother's last days on Earth and highlights major activities of my transition to life without Mom afterward. First it discusses Mom's home health care facility (home hospice) and life during that 30 months. Then, life at the nursing home afterward is detailed for the next 15 months until Mom's passing. Finally, my life after Mom's death—the major adjustment is chronicled. This chapter ends with a "journal entry" on May 2, 2008 detailing my state of life as it was on my 62nd birthday.

MOM'S HOME HOSPICE

By August of 2003 my mother's health had slipped badly. She was hospitalized and treated for various serious heart and kidney problems. After hospitalization she was discharged but came home an invalid, needing at first daytime nursing assistance, then, a little later round-the clock nursing monitoring.

The family 'circled the wagons'. Vince took over management of Mom's finances (investments) and from Cincinnati (where he lived) put together the game plan for Mom's home health care. He interviewed the certified nursing assistants (CNA's) and hired them. He also fired or let go those who did not work out. I was like the 'shop foreman'. I lived in the house with Mom, watched over the situation and paid the gals, reporting all problems to my brother. I also had additional duties. But these were limited as my disabilities did not permit full-scale involvement.

We had an assortment of CNA's ranging from rock solid full time professionals to part-time delights. On a disconcerting note we had one CNA who had murdered her husband and had spent time in the pen for it, and another who almost burned down the house accidently.

The daily routine was varying shifts 'round the clock' seven days a week. Aside from taking Mom to the bathroom and watching her health needs, the CNA's also cooked breakfast, lunch and supper for her, cleaned her apartment downstairs in the house, and entertained Mom, keeping her always in good spirits. I kept track of Mom's medications (17 pills each day in all), did all the shopping for food, medicine, household needs, etc. I drove Mom to dialysis twice per week and stayed with her until she was finished, or arranged to have an ambulance take and return her. Receiving lump sum distributions from Vince, I paid all Mom's bills and kept financial expense records. I also consulted on how to keep Mom's diet in line with doctor's orders buying only the 97 or so foods that she could eat safely.

Mom took well to the attention and care. She flourished in her role as CEO over the whole home health care operation and lived the life of the 'Queen of Sheba' with her attendants. For almost 2 1/2 years she lived a very happy life despite the fact that she knew that in the end she would not recover but would die.

I fared OK in the beginning. But, the added responsibilities caused growing 'job stress' even though the only pay I got was Mom's unconditional love and thanks and many free dinners (I ate with Mom nearly every night). After 30 months with only one one-week break I was physically and mentally exhausted.

Mom unfortunately fell finally. She never recovered from the fall and it simply became too expensive to keep her at home any more. Then, in January 2006 she went, at first with great resistance, to the nursing home. She had so wanted to die at home . . .

Vince put me in the hospital where I was treated for mental exhaustion and C.O.P.D. Physically I was a wreck, too. Discharged late in January I was sent to the nursing home too for a month of rehab. Thus, both Mom and I stayed together in separate rooms in the same place—Heartland of Marietta—for a little while yet.

HEARTLAND

Once convinced that the nursing home was the only safe place where she could be Mom adjusted gradually to being at Heartland, a modern nursing home and hospice located just north of Marietta in Devola which Vince found after researching the Internet. Heartland was a sprawling facility but properly staffed by friendly professionals and was really the perfect place for Mom given her present predicament.

Joining my mother at Heartland as a rehab patient after my discharge from Marietta Memorial Hospital in late January, I hunkered down for a month of skilled care.

Life at the nursing home centered around meal times, physical therapy, and roommates. There were two dining rooms: one for residents too ill to feed themselves and another for residents still able to feed themselves. Breakfast, lunch, and dinner were served punctually at the proper time by the staff on carts rolled out from the massive kitchen. Mom and I were both seated in the second dining room where we shared a table with other residents who were able to be yet a little conversant. Many conversations ensued both while I was yet a resident and after I was discharged and visited Mom regularly (daily) during her 15 month stay.

Physical therapy was by invitation. The PT specialist made it difficult for anybody to decline. Sessions lasted an hour or two and involved doing various exercises on the machines, playing with balls or doing other coordination tests. As a special treat sometimes the resident was allowed to eat a snack in the exercise area prepared in the small kitchen in the room at the end of the hall where the PT sessions were held.

Roommates varied. Mom's first roommate was mentally non-conversant. But she had other roommates who were quite bright and fun to be with, and who warmed up to her. My own roommate while I was there was a good hearted WWII veteran who learned from the PT people how to walk again. He was an amazing recovery.

In February I was discharged. But, I continued daily visits to Mom at Heartland and hospitals she was also occasionally sent until she died. We often ate together and shared the events of the day. Vince, Marge, and once in awhile Tim, Kathy and their son would visit too. Mom's friends from Vienna also came to visit her and have supper with her and me in the home's special residents' lounge.

Of special note was Mom's 96th birthday bash at the home. Quite a crowd of her family and friends came to be with Mom and share her birthday cake and trimmings.

Approaching her 97th birthday (March 2007), Mom's heart became very weak. She was transferred from resident care to hospice care. The family (Vince, Margie, Tim and I) had a small party for her the Saturday night before her Tuesday birthday. She died Monday afternoon. Her wake and funeral Mass were well attended.

THE TRANSITION

After my mother's death my brothers were concerned for me that her passing might destabilize my mind given that since my father's death in late '93 she had been my "significant other" more than anyone else. They pressed me to find a 'grief councilor' and also a regular therapist locally. Wanting to do this myself I was able to "sign up" three people to keep a check on me mentally. These were the pastor at the church, Carolyn Escandon, whom I met through following references, and a therapist at the local mental health agency. I also found a grief counseling group therapy session at the Wellness Center in Parkersburg. Thus, I assembled my 'team' to cushion the impact of my mother's passing and guide me to a new and better future.

Of course, I kept up regular contact with my two brothers by telephone, particularly with Vince in Cincinnati. But, they were after all distant from me geographically in case I needed 'immediate' help. My brothers and I stayed close otherwise however and I never developed a feeling of isolation that I feared might set in.

To keep busy, aside from the regular work out that staying healthy (with all of my maladies) required, I began to spend more and more effort in writing my books and other essays. I joined and participated in a Creative Writing or Journaling class at the Senior Center and spent much time reviewing my work with its other members.

Last but not least, I expanded my Faith-based activities seven fold developing over time a 'church family'. Through the pastor I became a member of the bulletin "Stuffing Group" at church where I met several new people. He also convinced me to join the Knights of Columbus where I met many more people. My friend of many years, Manuel Rodriguez, convinced me to sign up for Holy Hour weekly. As a result, I developed a prayer life (that had been lacking) before the Blessed Sacrament. I also joined in other parish activities as I was able.

Over the span of time from March 2007 to May 2008 I became known by many people in town and shared my writings with many of them. These efforts, coupled with the friendships I had built up over the years in Vienna and at my apartment complex provided a 'support group' that was the basis for staying and growing old in the Valley. I shelved contingency plans to move to Cincinnati to be close to 'family' at least for the time being.

BIRTHDAY 62

Soon, May 2008 arrived. And ever so quietly I slipped by the 'entrance to old age,' my 62nd birthday, on May second. Brother Vince, who was visiting while fixing up my mother's house for resale, took me out to supper on the first and second. And so my younger years ended and my 'older years' began.

I had arrived. But where?

JOURNAL ENTRY
MAY 2nd, 2008

At age 62 the state of my existence could be described as follows along four basic parameters:

MEDICALLY/PHYSICALLY: I am basically "a shipwreck". Disabled due to schizophrenia, add crippling diabetes (since 1992), osteoarthritis, and C.O.P.D. with chronic bronchitis and I am lucky I can still live outside a nursing home. I savor each day of living at home in my apartment, enjoying it as if it were my last. Half my awakened time it seems is spent either taking pills, shots, inhalers or procedures or going to the doctors and hospitals to have procedures and endless check-ups run there.

FINANCIALLY: I seem to be a 'disaster underway'. All my income is earmarked for taking care of living expenses. While I live on what I get for the majority of expenses, medical bills, particularly prescription drugs, 'blow me away'. Having been totally disabled for many years I have no significant savings to fall back on. But, I have a good relationship with an understanding family who bear me a sufficient-for-now amount of 'goodwill.'

MATERIALLY: Faring better in this department, while owning nothing of convertible-to-cash value except my 3 year old car, I own 'quite a bit of stuff'. My apartment is filled to the brim with utilitarian furniture, electronics, and heirlooms. Oil paintings (mostly done by Mom) and store-bought prints cover the walls. Drawers and other compartments are crammed full of smaller items. Office supplies are gradually being stockpiled in the den. I paid for or inherited all. I carry no debt.

SPIRITUALLY: This is my strongest suit—pretty good. I have a mostly positive view of the present and near future. My brothers and their families are 'good people' that are supportive of me. I have a few good friends—and no active enemies (that I know of). I am satisfied with my Church and above all, I am at peace with God—and He seems to be at peace with me.

REGRETS

A man who is not a veteran, never married or had children, and, to boot, only worked half of his adult life at a rate above "substantial gainful employment" one would think would be full of regrets as his time grows short and his return to his Maker approaches. In the Catholic Faith in which I was raised a man had three main duties: "to defend the flag of his country, to propagate the race, and to not be a burden to society". Politically, a person like me is "unelectable" to public office and is surrounded by in our society by whisperings and stigma. The common suspicion is that "he could have done better" . . .

Yet, if one looks at my life a little closer certain ameliorating circumstances emerge:

—Schizophrenia, guns and stress don't mix well. A heavily armed and uniformed schizophrenic soldier bent out of shape by stress is not a patriotic picture but rather the image of everyone's nightmares. I was unfit for military duty as the government so determined during the Vietnam War—and regardless of anything I thought or said at the time. I defended the flag in other less notable ways: working at defense plants, doing location work on defense plants later, and by paying taxes all the years I worked. I am satisfied that if America's enemies ever hang those who helped defend her I'll hang alongside the rest as "one fires the gun, the other loads it. All are equally 'guilty' . . ."

—Not everyone is suited for the married life. Schizophrenia by dimming the intellect in certain insidious ways for extended periods of time makes one most of the time a less than desirable husband and father. At any rate I never found an eligible woman who, knowing I was schizophrenic, sustained an interest in marrying me. I learned from life experience and group therapy sessions that there are far worse things than to go through life single. One of those worse things is to hook up with the wrong partner . . .

—Schizophrenia in my case seemed to be degenerative. While I was, with much extra effort, able to yet work during my younger years, I eventually deteriorated to the point of being a liability to my employer. At the end of the 1980's the doctors determined that I was unfit to work because of my disabilities. They continue to say so today. When doctors (eventually 32 of them) concur about that, employment becomes impossible as no hiring authority wants to hire a person who is unfit, lest they themselves are fired for putting people who can't perform into paying positions.

All of the above is not to say that my life was perfect. I burped and belched and occasionally even passed gas. Mistakes made were numerous as my judgment was often affected by my illness. But, I learned from most of my mistakes. So, while I sometimes made bad choices, I hardly ever made the same mistake twice. And, after awhile . . . the guard dogs quit barking.

One doesn't live to make bad choices—although mistakes are part of the learning process. Nevertheless, one lives for other reasons . . .

WHY DID I LIVE/WHY DO I CONTINUE TO LIVE?

Why did I live? Only God knows completely. But part of the reason was to do the things I did that occupied most of my waking hours. I lived to be a competitive student, a chemical worker, a professional geographer, a disabled entrepreneur and a care giver principally. I lived to relate as well as I could to my family and friends. And to find my way back into the Church at a later day.

Now why do I live? I am transitioning past my mother's death into "legitimate" retired living. Where to from here? There is no 'grand plan'. I'll take it one day at a time, and taking time out to smell the coffee in the mornings and the roses in the afternoons. Other times the doctors keep me busy taking care of my physical health and the Church keeps me active attending to mine and their spiritual needs. And I keep in touch with my family and friends . . .

WRAPPING UP . . .

It goes without saying that as full as my life was, it was not the life of a "great man". Millions of other men stand before me, higher in rank as "great men" before me. My life pales in comparison to the lives of both my brothers:

Vince, my older brother now retired as a chief engineer with GE, married well and had a large family (3 children) who in turn married and had children creating another generation of family. Reasonably wealthy, he and his wife spend their retirement years seeing to the needs of their abundant family.

Tim, my younger brother now also retired from being a chief engineer at Ford, also married well and reared one child. Tim amassed sizable wealth and spends his retirement years seeing to the needs of his teenage son and managing his upscale real estate holdings and furnishings.

Instead of being a "great man" I have told you the story of a "survivor" in a nearly life-long battle with schizophrenia and other problems related and unrelated. Currently somewhat victorious I spend my retirement days with my church family and other friends, my brothers and their families, and my books with their many rich memories.

And so Ron Doyle, the least of the Doyle boys from Livingston and Vienna, is now heard from . . .

THE END

APPENDIX

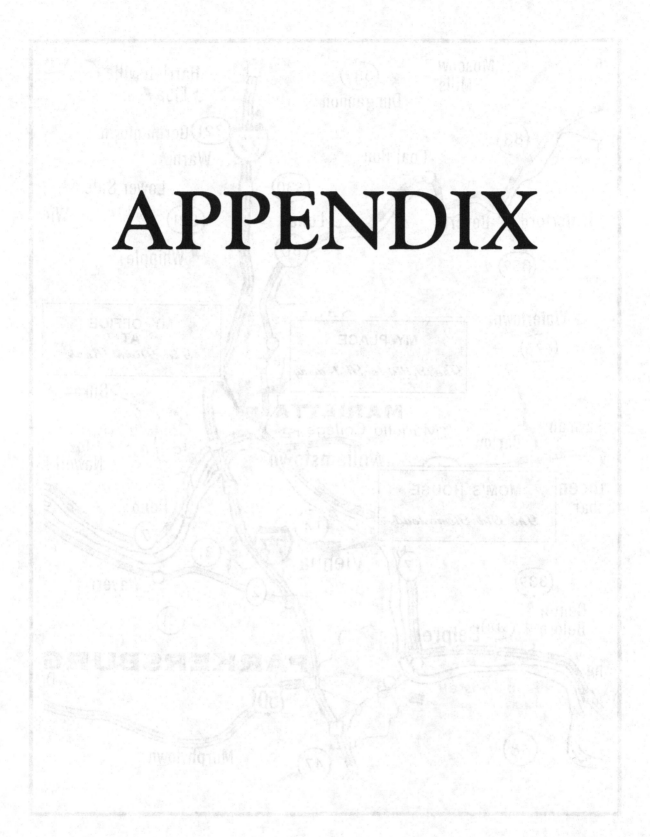

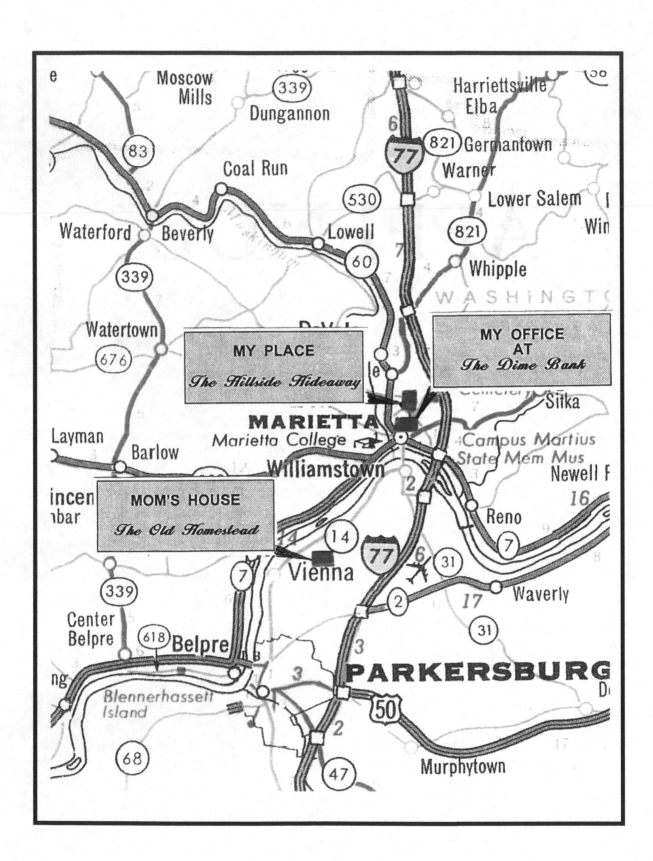

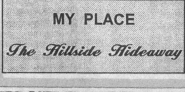

MY PLACE
The Hillside Hideaway

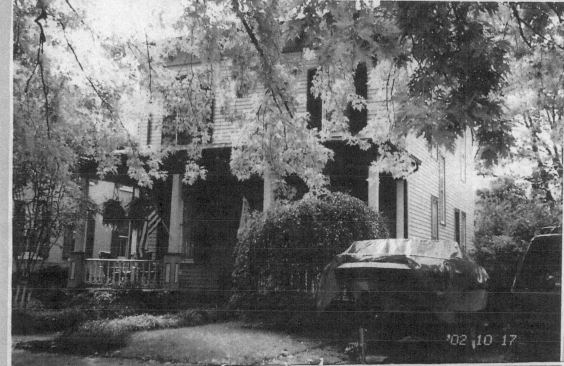

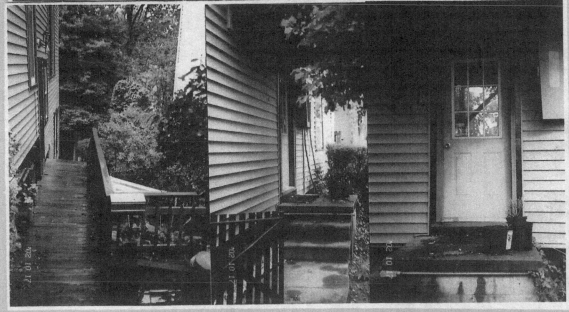

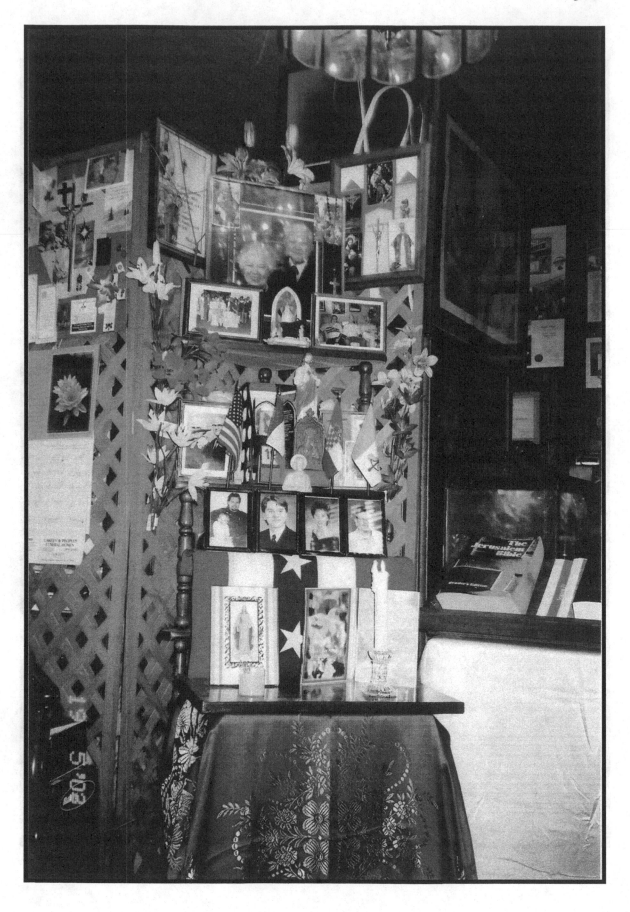

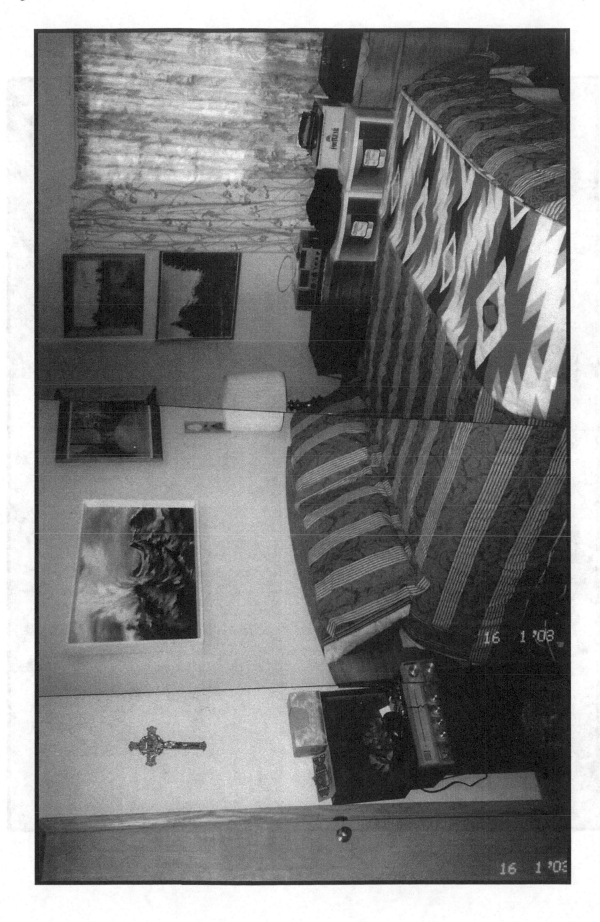

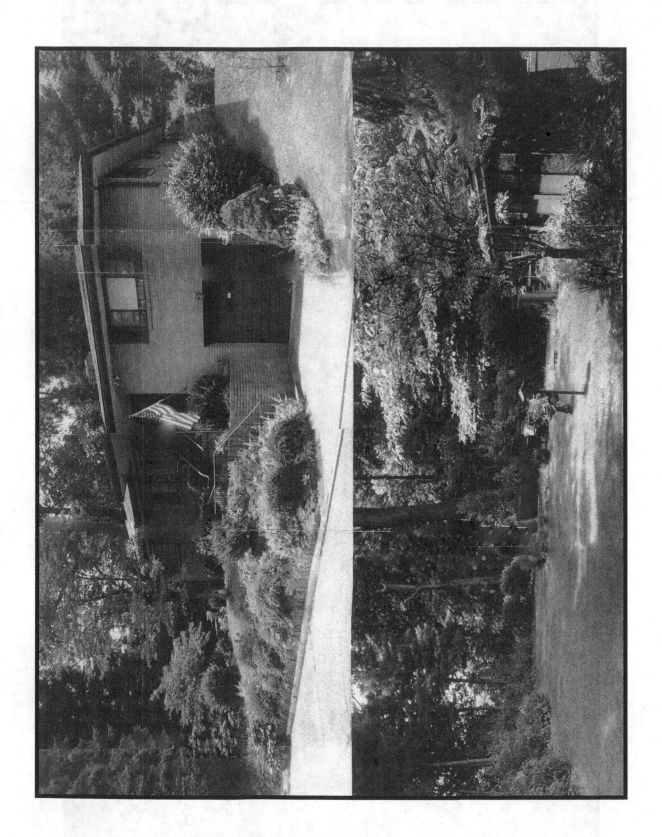

The Ohio (Department Of Mental Health)
Community Support Planning Council

LETTERS
2000-2003

323 1/2 Fifth Street
Marietta, OH 45750
Feb. 16, 2000

Mr. Terry Russell
NAMI-Ohio
747 East Broad Street
Columbus, OH 43205

Dear Terry:

You indicated to me very recently that a "consumer" position on the DMH Planning Council remains unfilled. I would like to be considered for that position. I think I have some insights and perspectives that may be useful and I want to be of assistance.

I was diagnosed with schizophrenia in 1968 while still in college. I managed to graduate, however, and went on into the work world where I stayed employed for 20 years until becoming totally disabled in 1987. Currently I'm recovering nicely and want to become more involved.

My more detailed qualifications include:

☞32 years personal experience combatting schizophrenia with the assistance of Ohio/WV mental health professionals (1968-Present);

☞Three college degrees:

> Bachelor of Arts (Geography), *The Ohio State University*, Columbus, OH (1969);
> Master of Arts (Geography), *The Ohio State University*, Columbus, OH (1971);
> Associate in Applied Business (Data Processing), *Washington Technical College*, Marietta, OH (1989);

☞20 years work experience as a professional geographer (1969-1989) including 14 years as a facility location consultant at *The Austin Company*, Cleveland, OH (1973-1987);

☞13 years of partial self-employment on my own (1987-Present);

☞2 years as a board member of NAMI/Washington County studying issues and practices in mental health (1998-Present);

☞No criminal convictions except minor traffic violations (Birth-Present).

I would welcome a telephone inquiry, a personal interview, or correspondence on this matter. I'm looking forward to hearing from you or the DMH.

Yours truly,

Ronald Frank Doyle

323 1/2 Fifth Street
Marietta, OH 45750
September 20, 2000

Mr. Terry Russell
NAMI-Ohio
747 East Broad Street
Columbus, OH 43205

Dear Terry:

You intervened to have me appointed very recently to a "consumer" position on the DMH Ohio
Community Support Planning Council. I have been told that I must be reelected in October
already as I was filling out the unexpired term of someone else. I would like to continue on in
that position as having been to just three meetings since my appointment I've just now have now
gotten oriented, and feel capable now of being some contribution in the future.

As stated in my last letter to you my qualifications include:

I was diagnosed with schizophrenia in 1968 while still in college. I managed to graduate,
however, and went on into the work world where I stayed employed for 20 years until becoming
totally disabled in 1987. Currently I'm recovering nicely and want to become more involved.

My more detailed qualifications include:

☞32 years personal experience combatting schizophrenia with the assistance of
Ohio/WV mental health professionals (1968-Present);

☞Three college degrees:

> Bachelor of Arts (Geography), *The Ohio State University*,
> Columbus, OH (1969);
> Master of Arts (Geography), *The Ohio State University*, Columbus,
> OH (1971);
> Associate in Applied Business (Data Processing), *Washington
> Technical College*, Marietta, OH (1989);

☞20 years work experience as a professional geographer (1969-1989) including 14
years as a facility location consultant at *The Austin Company*, Cleveland, OH
(1973-1987);

☞13 years of partial self-employment on my own (1987-Present);

☞2 years as a board member of NAMI/Washington County studying issues and
practices in mental health (1998-Present);

☞No criminal convictions except minor traffic violations (Birth-Present).

I would welcome your continued support. Enclosed is my application sent on to the DMH.

Yours truly,

Ronald Frank Doyle

323 1/2 Fifth Street
Marietta, OH 45750
September 20, 2000

Grisetta Griffin, Asst. Chief
OHIO DEPARTMENT OF MENTAL HEALTH
Office of Consumer Services
30 East Broad Street, 8th Floor
Columbus, OH 43266-0414

Dear Ms. Griffin:

Enclosed please find applications for two Planning Council candidates for the October nominations. If you have any questions or need more information please call me at (740) 373-0209 daytime.

Thanks for your consideration in advance.

Yours truly,

Ron Doyle
Consumer
East Southern District

323 1/2 Fifth Street
Marietta, OH 45750
September 27, 2000

Greg Moody
Ohio Family and Children First
17 South High Street, Ste 550
Columbus, OH 43215

Dear Greg:

In answer to questions 2 through 4 on the sheet entitled "Identifying Ohio's Commitments to Child Well Being" I address the following:

I am currently a member of the Ohio Community Support Planning Council just now becoming informed and proactive in council affairs. Besides being a consumer I am also the uncle of a boy who has been diagnosed bi-polar. He is 10 and lives in another state with my brother and his wife.

All of the commitments listed support my efforts to improve child well being. But these commitments need to be backed up by money and correct procedures as I'm sure you are aware.

Judging from my brother's experience with my bi-polar nephew it would appear that the State of Ohio is moving in the right direction with alternative education, infant mental health, and the red flags program but I see a need for more assertive community treatment (ACT) for children with mental health problems and support for their parents. My brother, who has financial resources, is nevertheless almost at wit's end by the problems my nephew creates and experiences due to his bi-polar condition. The State of Ohio in helping Ohio's children should put more pressure on physicians and/or treating agencies to provide more on-call advice and assistance particularly to the parents, and support groups to them to hash out with one another and with professionals ways and means of coping. Currently, even with the financial resources, advice is given by a treating psychiatrist for an hour or so each month. Then the boy and the parents are left alone to cope with one situation after another. More back-up is needed and ought to be available (if necessary funded for those who don't have money).

In other matters, I find the medicine being developed by the drug companies is getting better and better. The State of Ohio would do well to encourage even more medical research providing perhaps tax and other incentives where appropriate.

Thank you for your inquiry of my perspective.

Yours truly,

Ronald F. Doyle
OCSPC-Consumer
East Southern District

323 1/2 Fifth Street
Marietta, OH 45750
October 16, 2000

Mr. Terrence Dalton
Comm. Support Services
150 Cross Street
Akron, OH 44311

RE: Ohio Community Support Planning Council Business;
A forensic matter concerning adults: mental health courts.

Dear Terry:

It appears that mental health courts for mentally ill non-violent offenders is an idea whose time has come. But while several urban areas in Ohio have these courts, demand and county budgets are likely too low to afford this progress in most of rural Ohio including the East Southern District which I represent. Yet, it is the intention of the ODMH that all Ohioans have accessibility to whatever services are offered. Justice demands that people living in rural Ohio have availability to mental health courts too.

I think the Planning Council should propose a regionalization plan of mental health courts to cover the rest of the State, grouping counties together in a region large enough to financially afford and where demand is high enough to warrant a mental health court. Perhaps a circuit judge approach could be used where the regional judge holds court first in one county then in another then in the next until the region of smaller counties is served. Part-time mental health courts could also be utilized but then the expertise of the regular judge doubling as a part-time mental health court judge may be overtaxed. At any rate, a mental health court in every small county need not be if regional courts can be established. As one of our speakers pointed out recently, "You can buy quite a bit of case management for the cost of paying a judge."

The literature points out that 35-40% of adults with SMI ultimately come at odds with the criminal justice system. Let's forward the idea of regional mental health courts to cover the rural counties of Ohio on the same basis as the urban counties so all Ohioans can avail themselves of this protection.

Yours truly,

Ronald F. Doyle
Consumer-East Southern District
Ohio Community Support Planning Council

323 1/2 Fifth Street
Marietta, OH 45750
October 29, 2000

Mr. Terrence Dalton
Comm. Support Services
150 Cross Street
Akron, OH 44311

RE: WE WOULD LIKE YOUR FEEDBACK

Dear Terry:

Here are my answers to your questions:

1. Specific draft recommendations for a new strategic management plan to meet the needs of people with mental illness are still being developed. However, the Commission's plan is to make recommendations in four categories: improving access, effective treatment, system design and finances. Do these catagories seem inclusive of the areas where work needs to be done? Is anything missing? What are two or three specific items within any of these catagories that you feel the Commission must address?

The categories seem to be adequate. Within each category the Commission should at least address the following:

Improving access: Rural counties should be served on the same basis as urban counties where possible. (i. e. mental health courts for rural counties ought to be established, other urban services should include rural counties in their catchment areas.)

Effective treatment: Treating agencies should be more responsible for enrolling relatives in support groups and in creating support groups for the SMI people. They should be more responsible for helping relatives as well as SMI's cope. It is far too easy for SMI's to become penniless and isolated. More PACT's and ACT's are needed.)

System design: The Oakwood (forensic) facility should remain open. There needs to be a place to receive criminally insane other than prison.

Finances: There needs to be a higher budget overall. Particularly I've noticed in this area that case workers seem to be in short supply.

2. In order, what are the three most important issues facing the public mental health system today and into the near future?

As I see it from a review of the literature and from my perspective: 1) more money to service an expanding caseload; 2) rural vs. urban parity of services; 3) reduce prison bound SMI population.

3. Have you heard about the Commission before? How can the Commission be more responsive to your need for information about the Commission's work?

I heard about the Commission through the Planning Council. The Commission has adequately responded to my need for information thus far.

4. Following relase of the Commission's final report, what next steps would you like to see regarding discussion and implementation of the recommendations?

I would like to see the Planning Council discuss and the Director implement the recommendations that the Plannning Council finds valid and worthwhile.

Yours truly,

Ronald F. Doyle
Consumer-East Southern District
Ohio Community Support Planning Council

323 1/2 Fifth Street
Marietta, Ohio 45750
August 2, 2001

Mr. Patrick Duffy
5930 Heisley Road
Mentor, OH 44060

RE: Ohio's Death Penalty as pertains to the Mentally Ill

Dear Mr. Duffy:

Following please find the most compelling arguments I can think of against capital punishment for the mentally ill criminals of Ohio...

THOUGHTS ON THE DEATH PENALTY
FOR MENTALLY ILL CRIMINALS IN OHIO

1. West Virginia, a neighboring state to Ohio, has <u>no death penalty at all</u>. Gov. Hulett Smith (Dem) abolished it in the 1960's and it has never been reinstated. The state has a very low crime rate despite this and the existance of much poverty too! It also saves the state money because it is usually cheaper to keep a person in prison for life than to execute him/her due to the high cost of the appeals process.

2. A death sentence is meant to serve as an example to others not to commit the capital crime. But, in the case of a mentally ill person that person usually is not understanding much when he commits the crime. A mental disorder most often is more dimming of the intellect than is temporary insanity in crimes of passion...

3. Because of a lack of cognizant responsibility, Ohio doesn't execute children nor, I believe, the mentally retarded. The mentally ill suffer from the same kind of diminished responsibility.

4. Mental illness is a punishment of sorts in and of itself. How can we feel right in adding to what God and nature have delivered? And life in prison or better in a hospital for the criminally insane is afterall not a light penalty.

5. A brain disorder in that it causes **dementia** is quite understandable to an intelligent person. Of course the mentally ill very often do not realize the boundaries of sensible talk and behavior! To protect public safety some need to be locked up, some permanently, but mental illness should never be a <u>terminal</u> experience.

In closing, the majority of the Council feels that justice in this matter is better served by extending the benefit of the doubt, compassion, and leniency to the mentally ill.

I hope this is helpful to you in writing the draft of the Council's letter. I may be contacted on my cell phone afternoons at (304) 481-0605 or at my mother's house early evenings at (304) 295-6060.

Regards,

Ron Doyle
Consumer-East Southern District

323 1/2 Fifth Street
Marietta, OH 45750
August 17, 2002

Mr. Terrence Dalton
Comm. Support Services
150 Cross Street
Akron, OH 44311

RE: Ohio Community Support Planning Council Business;
Resignation of Planning Council Member.

Dear Terry:

I hereby resign my position on the Planning Council as of December 31, 2002.
I will <u>not</u> be a candidate for reelection in October.

As you may know, my principal occupation nowadays is looking after the needs of my 92 year old mother. Her health is such that I am becoming increasingly uncomfortable to leave her alone for entire days while I attend the Council meetings in far away Columbus. And sitters are hard to find. But, also I am uncomfortable with seeking a leadership position in the mental health politics of the Southern Region which I represent. My principal contacts down here were through NAMI/Washington County, and with that organization now defunct, I am left to spend time and money reaching out to unfamiliar leadership circles. I don't feel up to the task and can't commit to take the time due to serving my mother's sporatic but often urgent needs. So, I've decided to leave the position open to someone else who can be a better representative.

I've enjoyed my time on the Council and have learned a great deal. I've found though that Council members seem to grasp well the problem without much comment from me. I endorse the Council's efforts to focus attention (and hopefully more money) on meeting the needs of the mentally ill and wish the Council success in these endeavors.

I remain committed to doing what I should to help your efforts.

Sincerely yours,

Ronald F. Doyle
Consumer-East Southern District
Ohio Community Support Planning Council

PRESCRIPTION DRUGS AT A DISCOUNT
FOR SENIORS AND DISABLED
ON MEDICARE

There are a number of prescription drug discount cards on the market. This one if FREE, however, and NEW. It promises a lot! So far, I'm still trying to get this card, but you may have better luck. Be very careful to specify that you or the applicant is not on any public or private drug assistance plan.

FROM: RON DOYLE
SOUTHERN DISTRICT

State of Ohio
Bob Taft, Governor

Department of Mental Health
Michael F. Hogan, Ph.D., Director

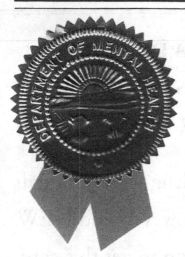

Certificate of Appreciation

Presented to

Ronald Doyle

in recognition of your contributions to the work of the Ohio Department of Mental Health as a member of the Ohio Community Support Planning Council. Your dedication, leadership and advocacy efforts have helped Ohio lead the nation in the development of consumer-centered service delivery systems. Your assistance in promoting increased access to integrated and supportive consumer-based systems which provide consumer voice and choice, culturally competent services, consumer quality review, advance directives and consumer protections is much appreciated. Thank you for your commitment to improving the quality of life for Ohio's children and adults with mental illness.

Presented this 14th day of December, 2002.

Michael F. Hogan, Ph.D., Director
Ohio Department of Mental Health

323 1/2 Fifth Street
Marietta, OH 45750
December 31, 2002

Michael F. Hogan, Ph.D
Director
Ohio Department of Mental Health
Eighth Floor, Rhodes Office Tower
30 East Broad Street
Columbus, OH 43215-3430

Re: Planning Council business

Dear Dr. Hogan:

I am in receipt of a Certicate of Appreciation presented to me in my absence
on December 14, 2002. While the threat of inclement weather prevented me
from attending my final meeting I want to thank you for recognizing my
efforts to serve you, the State, and the mentallly ill of Ohio. I considered it
an honor to serve as a consumer on the Ohio Community Support Planning
Council and hope I helped the situation some. I have now withdrawn to serve
full time the needs of my 92 year old mother who lives directly across the
river from Marietta in West Virginia.

While most of what I had to contribute was said at the Council meetings a
couple of loose ends still need addressed to you:

Rural Mental Health Courts. Mental health courts are a good idea. I support
just about anything that would get the mentally ill out of regular criminal
courts and protect us from runaway juries with their "let's-hang-em-and-go-
get-lunch" attitude that is particularly prevalent in rural Ohio. I proposed a
regional mental health court scheme for the state (See attached) that would
make it possible to cover rural counties as well. (Local people here **hate** drug
addicts and alchoholics. The mentally ill carry of strong stigma too but at
least it is generally recognized that they are not *doing* something to cause their
inappropriate behavior...)

The Death Penalty. I still would like to see the Council and ODMH push for
an end to the death penalty for mentally ill criminals. The Council did pass
such a resolution but before a letter could be sent the events of 9/11/01
stunned the nation. People thought these criminals once caught would be
found to be mentally ill and sentiment supported the emotional counter
argument that a jury should be allowed to decide appropriate punishment for
bizarre criminal acts. The terrorists are not mentally ill. Evil exists quite
aside from mental illness. And the truly mentally ill have diminished
responsibility for their actions.

<u>Prescription Drug Costs</u>.   These costs simply need attacked by as many effective means as possible, at least for people working or disabled who are covered only by Medicare or have no insurance at all!   I am an example. My Risperdal, the only effective treatment I have found for my schizophrenia, costs $330/month---and with other prescription drugs I take my typical monthly drug bill exceeds $710/month!   That's more than 50% of my SSDI payment. Were I to work that would be a huge bite out of my earnings and with schizophrenia often corporate insurance companies won't cover me.   I am not alone.   Drug costs potentially **cancel out** the good done by the most ambitious government and employer originated assistance programs for the mentally ill. (Fortunately for me, some of the drug companies have patient assistance programs for low income people and I am receiving substantial assistance through these private efforts.   But, I hold my breath and pray each time I must reapply, and that is frequently.)

<u>The Need for Information</u>.   Families of those striken with mental illness have a chronic need for all sorts of information.   Doctors, usually with bulging case loads, are simply not able to meet these needs.   The 1-800 number for the ODMH appropriately staffed would be a great help to guide both family and consumers through this difficult adjustment.

Once again, thank you for the opportunity to put forth needs I've noticed.

Yours truly,

Ronald F. Doyle
OCSPC-Consumer
East Southern District

Ohio Department of Mental Health

30 East Broad Street
Columbus, Ohio 43266-0414

Phone: (614) 466-2596
TDD: (614) 752-9696
Fax: (614) 752-9453

February 6, 2003

Ronald F. Doyle
OCSPC-Consumer
East Southern District
323½ Fifth Street
Marietta, OH 45750

Dear Mr. Doyle,

Thank you for your letter of January 24, 2003. Although we will miss your participation
on the Planning Council, your continued advocacy efforts will make a difference in the
community and across the state. Your personal prioritization of "family first" by caring
for an aging family member deserves recognition.

You raise a number of concerns in your letter about the mental health system. These
major issues require ongoing attention from the mental health program and policy
perspective. Since these issues are facing Ohio as well as most other states, our local and
national focus continues to address improvements in the mental health system for
consumers. Our first priority is to listen to you and other consumers. Through that
listening, we strive to understand. Your issues reflect relevant concerns including mental
health courts, stigma, prescription drug costs, and communication of information. In
addressing these, our goal is to clearly support Recovery.

We appreciate your work on the Planning Council and your efforts to improve the mental
health system. To assure that we effectively utilize the information you have sent to us,
Judy Wortham Wood, Deputy Director is willing to meet with you for further discussion.
As a consumer and a Planning Council member, you are important to us. You may call
Judy or her assistant, Susan Watts at 466-4124.

Sincerely,

Michael F. Hogan, Ph.D.
Director

cc: Judy Wortham Wood, Deputy Director
    Grisetta Griffin, Manager, Consumer Services
    Sherry Boyd, Consumer Services

Accredited by the Joint Commission on Accreditation of Healthcare Organizations

An Equal Opportunity Employer/Provider

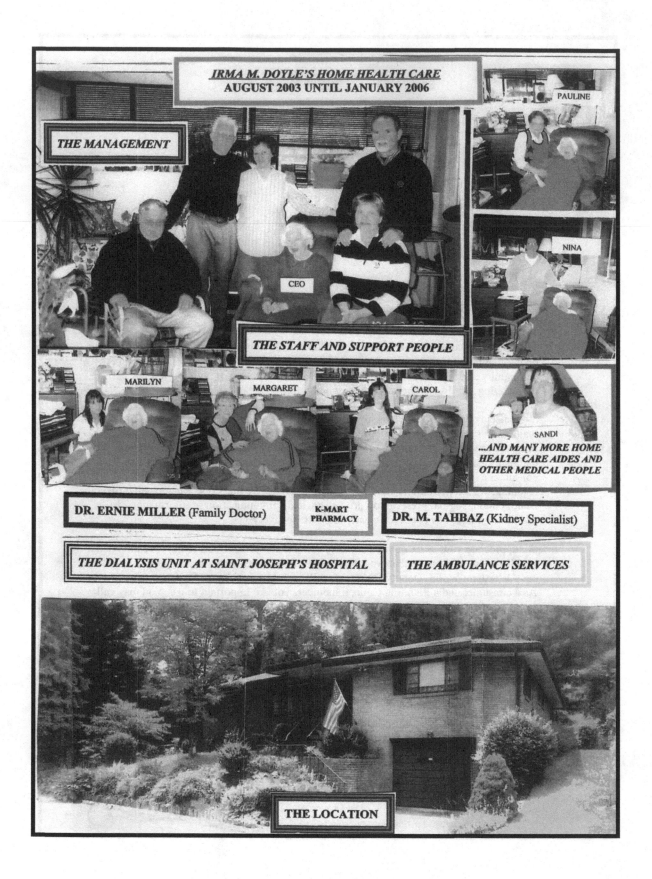

IRMA M. DOYLE'S HOME HEALTH CARE
AUGUST 2003 UNTIL JANUARY 2006

PAULINE

THE MANAGEMENT

CEO

NINA

THE STAFF AND SUPPORT PEOPLE

MARILYN

MARGARET

CAROL

SANDI

...AND MANY MORE HOME HEALTH CARE AIDES AND OTHER MEDICAL PEOPLE

DR. ERNIE MILLER (Family Doctor)

K-MART PHARMACY

DR. M. TAHBAZ (Kidney Specialist)

THE DIALYSIS UNIT AT SAINT JOSEPH'S HOSPITAL

THE AMBULANCE SERVICES

THE LOCATION

Irma M. Doyle

Irma Milisits Doyle, 96, of Vienna died March 19, 2007, at the St. Josephs Hospital.

She was born March 20, 1910, in New York, N.Y., the daughter of the late Frank and Mitzi Transits Milisits.

Doyle

She graduated from St. Marys High School in Scranton, Pa. She married Vincent "Vinnie" Doyle in 1939 and made Livingston, N.J., their home until 1956 when the family moved to Vienna. She was active in the Parkersburg Art League and along with her husband was a founding member of the St. Michael's Catholic Church in Vienna.

She is survived by her children, Vincent L. Doyle and his wife, Margaret Smith Doyle, of West Chester, Ohio, Ronald F. Doyle of Marietta and Timothy K. Doyle and his wife, Kathleen Cole Doyle, of Northville, Mich.; four grandchildren; and one great-granddaughter.

She was preceded in death by her loving husband, Vincent "Vinnie" Doyle; and one brother, Edgar F. Milisits. There will be a Memorial Mass 10 a.m. Friday at the St. Michael's Catholic Church in Vienna, with Father Steve Joseph officiating. Burial will be in the Mt. Carmel Cemetery. Visitation will be 4-8 p.m. Thursday at the Leavitt Funeral Home in Parkersburg, with a Christian Wake service at 6 p.m.

Memorial donations may be made to the donors favorite charity.

Online condolences may be made at www.leavittfuneralhome.com

Leavitt Funeral Home
Parkersburg, WV Belpre, OH

© Lasercraft Inc., N. Co., MO   Made in U.S.A.

<u>Irma M. Doyle</u>, mother of Ron Doyle of Vienna, WV, passed away March 19ᵗʰ. She had recently been a patient at Heartland of Marietta. Our prayers are with Ron and his family and we offer them our sympathy. May Mrs. Doyle now enjoy <u>eternal happiness.</u>

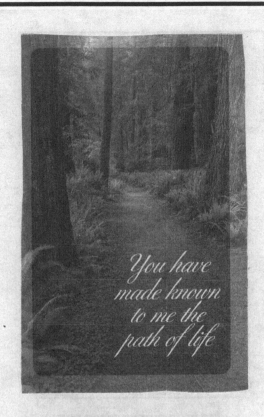

You have made known to me the path of life

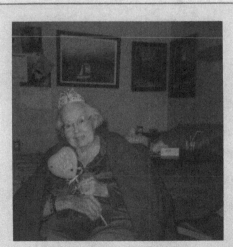

Valentines Day 2007

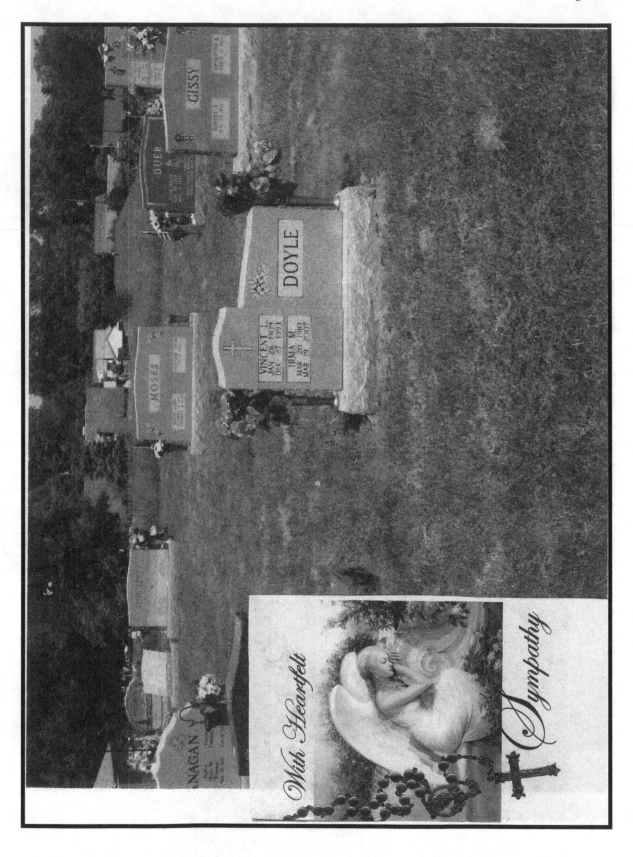

EPILOGUE

MAY 2, 2011

Since completing this series of books in 2008, life has continued to unfold. After a brief period of retired near-bliss, the other shoe fell and I met with severe health reversals associated with kidney failure. I was put on dialysis machinery pending finding a match for a kidney transplant. These and other medical costs consumed my entire inheritance as well as what little savings I had. And I went through the stages I needed to go through to qualify for Medicaid.

My life nowadays, besides a rare appearance at Catholic fraternal and religious events, consists of dialysis every Monday, Wednesday, and Friday and the recovery afterward. I live for the weekends and for Tuesday and Thursday when I don't have dialysis. Life on my days off is still good, however.

One final comment needs to be made as the twofold reason I wrote these books:

First, I wrote the books to dispel certain myths about schizophrenics; namely, that people with schizophrenia all come from poor backgrounds, were unloved by their parents, and have no worth as people. Also to promote the realization among the mentally ill and their families that a diagnosis of "mental illness" is not the end of the road. Life goes on. If careful, memories at the end of your life will be more positive than negative. Keep trying. While the efforts of a mentally ill person will most probably not be successful in a worldly sense, the fact that one made the efforts will be a source of satisfaction in the end. Be careful.

And a final message comes from me to all no matter what the adverse circumstances of your life are: "Hang in there! Better days are coming . . ." as my father often said to me.

Your comments and donations if so moved may be sent to:

Ron Doyle
C/o Doyle and Associates, Inc.
P.O. Box 2135
Marietta, OH 45750